Privacy and Confidentiality in Mental Health Care

Privacy and Confidentiality in Mental Health Care

edited by

John J. Gates, Ph.D.
The Carter Center Mental Health Program
Atlanta, Georgia

and

Bernard S. Arons, M.D.
The Center for Mental Health Services
Rockville, Maryland

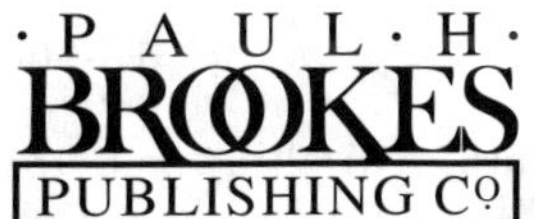

Baltimore • London • Toronto • Sydney

Paul H. Brookes Publishing Co.
Post Office Box 10624
Baltimore, Maryland 21285-0624

www.brookespublishing.com

Typeset by Brushwood Graphics, Baltimore, Maryland.
Manufactured in the United States of America by
Versa Press, East Peoria, Illinois.

The case studies described in this book are based on the authors' actual
experiences. Individuals' names have been changed and identifying
details have been altered to protect their confidentiality.

Library of Congress Cataloging-in-Publication Data

Privacy and confidentiality in mental health care / edited by John J. Gates
and Bernard S. Arons.
       p.   cm.
   Includes bibliographical references and index.
   ISBN 1-557-66-426-9
   1. Psychiatric records—Access control.   2. Psychiatric records—Access
control—United States.   I. Gates, John J.   II. Arons, Bernard S.
RC455.2.M38 P73   1999
362.2—dc21   99-045960

British Library Cataloguing in Publication data are available from the
British Library.

Contents

About the Editors vii
About the Contributors ix
Foreword   *Rosalynn Carter* xiii
Foreword   *Tipper Gore* xvii
Acknowledgments xxiii

1   Introduction
    John J. Gates and Bernard S. Arons 1

2   Consumers' Perspective of Confidentiality
    and Health Records
    Jean Campbell 5

3   Families' Perspectives on Confidentiality
    in the Treatment of Mental Illness
    Harriet P. Lefley 33

4   Privacy Issues in Child Mental
    Health Services
    Gary B. Melton 47

5   Clinical Issues in Mental Health Care
    Marcia Kraft Goin 71

6   Legal and Ethical Issues in Protecting the
    Privacy of Behavioral Health Care Information
    John Petrila 91

7   Will Technology Help or Hurt in the
    Struggle for Health Privacy?
    Robert Gellman 127

8   Confidentiality and HIV/AIDS:
    Professional Challenges
    Robert L. Barret 157

9   Confidentiality of Alcohol and Other Drug
    Patient Records
    Paul N. Samuels 173

vi   Contents

10   The Importance of Privacy and Limits
      to Privacy
      John J. Gates and Judy Fitzgerald 193

Appendix   State Mental Health Confidentiality
            Law Provisions
            John Petrila 219

Index 233

About the Editors

John J. Gates, Ph.D., Director, The Carter Center Mental Health Program, One Copenhill, 453 Freedom Parkway, Atlanta, GA 30307

Since 1993, Dr. Gates has implemented the initiatives of The Carter Center Mental Health Task Force, chaired by former U.S. First Lady Rosalynn Carter. Dr. Gates has worked closely with national and international organizations to foster and support mental health activities worldwide.

Through the Mental Health Program's annual symposia, forum, and journalism fellowships, Dr. Gates oversees efforts to identify major mental health issues, convene action-oriented meetings, and develop initiatives to reduce stigma and discrimination against those who experience mental illness. In addition, he works closely with Mrs. Carter on various key projects, including the International Committee of Women Leaders for Mental Health—a coalition of nearly 40 first ladies, royalty, and heads of state working to improve the status of mental health worldwide.

Prior to joining The Carter Center, Dr. Gates served several key roles in the Georgia Department of Human Resources, including Director of the State Mental Health, Mental Retardation and Substance Abuse Agency. He was also superintendent of the largest state-owned mental hospital in Georgia, successfully directing its efforts to be accredited for the first time in its 143-year history. He completed requirements in both the clinical and school psychology programs of Florida State University and was awarded a doctorate in 1966.

Dr. Gates serves on the boards of the Rosalynn Carter Institute for Human Development, the National Mental Health Association, and the World Federation for Mental Health. With several of his Carter Institute board members, Dr. Gates co-authored *Caring and Competent Caregivers* (University of Georgia Press, 1998). He is a member of the American Psychological Association, a fellow of the Georgia Psychological Association, and an honorary life member of the Mental Health Association of Georgia. Dr. Gates has also served as consultant and group facilitator to many organizations, including federal and state agencies, parties in class-action lawsuits, consumer and advocacy groups, and hospital and community service providers.

Bernard S. Arons, M.D., Director, The Center for Mental Health Services (CMHS), Substance Abuse and Mental Health Services Administration, U.S. Department of Health and Human Services, 5600 Fishers Lane, Room 15-505, Rockville, MD 20857

Dr. Arons began his career as a psychiatrist at St. Elizabeth's Hospital in Washington, D.C., where he treated patients with serious mental illnesses. He also served as an administrator while there and both taught and trained psychiatric residents, medical and social work students, and college volunteers. In 1980, Dr. Arons was appointed Director of the Dixon Implementation Office for St. Elizabeth's Hospital and was responsible for the hospital's major clinical care and deinstitutionalization plan. He then became the Chief Clinical Advisor and provided direction to the medical, nursing, psychology, and social work staffs.

In 1986, Dr. Arons joined a division of the National Institute of Mental Health as Associate Director for Mental Health Financing. In 1989, he was selected as a Legislative Fellow in the U.S. Congress. As one of the federal government managers/scientists to experience and contribute to the legislative process, he served as a legislative assistant to the Chair of the Health Subcommittee of the Ways and Means Committee of the U.S. House of Representatives.

Dr. Arons was tapped in early 1993 as an advisor on mental health issues to Mrs. Tipper Gore in the Office of the Vice President. Subsequently, as chair of the Mental Health and Substance Abuse Working Group Cluster of the President's Task Force on National Health Care Reform, Dr. Arons had an historic opportunity to focus the United States of America's attention on the importance of the inclusion of mental health care in a reformed national health care system.

In November 1993, Dr. Arons was appointed Director of the CMHS, a component of the Substance Abuse and Mental Health Services Administration. The CMHS is charged with providing national leadership in mental health services and policies.

Dr. Arons continues to teach and practice psychiatry at the Center for Mental Health, Inc., a private, nonprofit clinic in the District of Columbia. He also serves as a clinical professor of psychiatry on the faculty of Georgetown University School of Medicine.

Dr. Arons is a graduate of Oberlin College and Case Western Reserve University School of Medicine. His presentations and publications include articles on people with serious mental illnesses and health care reform. His membership on numerous boards, societies, and committees speaks to his ceaseless commitment to consumers of mental health services and their families.

About the Contributors

Robert L. Barret, Ph.D., Professor of Counselor Education, Department of Human Services, College of Education and Allied Professions, University of North Carolina at Charlotte, Charlotte, NC 28223

Dr. Barret is a psychologist in Charlotte, North Carolina. He began working with patients with HIV in 1984 and very quickly became a trainer of others seeking expertise in this work. He has served as a senior faculty member on two HIV/AIDS training projects under the auspices of the American Psychological Association. He is the co-editor of *Ethical Issues in HIV-Related Psychotherapy*, to be published by the American Psychological Association.

Jean Campbell, Ph.D., Research Assistant Professor, Missouri Institute of Mental Health: A Center for Policy, Research, and Training, University of Missouri School of Medicine–Columbia, 5400 Arsenal Street, St. Louis, MO 63139

Dr. Campbell is a Research Assistant Professor in the School of Psychiatry, University of Missouri School of Medicine–Columbia, and Director of the program in consumer studies and training at the Missouri Institute of Mental Health in St. Louis. She is currently Principal Investigator of a national cross-site study of consumer-operated service programs funded by the Substance Abuse and Mental Health Services Administration. An internationally known speaker and author, she leads the effort to promote the mental health consumer perspective in research and data issues.

Judy Fitzgerald, M.S.W., Associate Director, Human Systems and Outcomes, Inc., 2107 Delta Way, Tallahassee, FL 32303

Ms. Fitzgerald earned a master's degree in social work with a concentration in public policy from the University of Georgia in 1994. Since that time, she has worked for The Carter Center Mental Health Program and played an active role in local and state mental health advocacy efforts.

Robert Gellman, J.D., Privacy and Information Policy Consultant, 431 Fifth Street, SE, Washington, DC 20003

Mr. Gellman is a privacy and information policy consultant in Washington, D.C., and a graduate of the Yale Law School.

Marcia Kraft Goin, M.D., Ph.D., Clinical Professor of Psychiatry, University of Southern California School of Medicine, 1127 Wilshire Boulevard, Suite 1115, Los Angeles, CA 90017

Dr. Goin is Director of Psychiatric Residency Education in the Adult Psychiatric Outpatient Department of the Los Angeles County/ University of Southern California Medical Center. She is past chairperson of the American Psychiatric Association's Committee on Confidentiality, has testified before Congress on confidentiality legislation, and is an elected member of the Board of Trustees of the American Psychiatric Association.

Harriet P. Lefley, Ph.D., Professor, Department of Psychiatry and Behavioral Sciences, University of Miami School of Medicine, Post Office Box 016960, Miami, FL 33101

Dr. Lefley is Professor of Psychiatry and Behavioral Sciences at the University of Miami School of Medicine, a licensed psychologist, and active in advocacy for people with mental illness. She has published 7 books and more than 100 articles and book chapters dealing with cultural, community, and family issues in mental health. For more than 15 years, Dr. Lefley has led weekly support groups for families of people with major mental illness during which issues of confidentiality frequently arise.

Gary B. Melton, Ph.D., Director, Institute for Families in Society, University of South Carolina, 937 Assembly Street, Columbia, SC 29208

The author of more than 250 publications, Dr. Melton has written extensively on child and family policy. Much of his recent work has focused on the application of international human rights law to such issues. A past president of the American Psychology-Law Society and the American Psychological Association (APA) Division of Child, Youth, and Family Services, Dr. Melton has received distinguished contribution awards from two divisions of APA, Psi Chi, and Prevent Child Abuse America.

John Petrila, J.D., LL.M., Chair and Professor, Department of Mental Health Law and Policy, Louis de la Parte Florida Mental Health Institute, University of South Florida, 13301 Bruce B. Downs Boulevard, Tampa, FL 33612

Mr. Petrila is Chair of the Department of Mental Health Law and Policy at the Louis de la Parte Florida Mental Health Institute. He publishes and lectures frequently on mental disability law issues. He was formerly General Counsel to the New York State Office of Mental Health.

Paul N. Samuels, J.D., Director, The Legal Action Center, 153 Waverly Place, 8th Floor, New York, NY 10014

Mr. Samuels began work as a staff attorney at The Legal Action Center in 1979 and became Director/President in 1992. The Legal Action Center is a nonprofit, public interest law and policy organization that advocates on behalf of people with histories of drug and alcohol dependence, HIV/AIDS, or criminal records as well as for sound public policies in these areas. Mr. Samuels is a graduate of Harvard College and Columbia University Law School.

Foreword

We Americans have long considered privacy a core value of our personal freedom. Advances in technology regarding the storage and transfer of information and increasing demands for access to information have led us to be very concerned about the erosion of privacy. These developments require us to think differently about the notion of privacy in our modern society. We now question the ability to adequately protect our personal information, and, as a society, we are challenged to balance historical individual rights with legitimate claims for access to information.

Nowhere is this balance more difficult to achieve than in the privacy of health information. Dramatic changes in the organization, financing, and delivery of health care have resulted in sophisticated and complicated health systems that sometimes confuse and overwhelm consumers. This complexity is magnified when discussing mental health information. Although confidentiality is a cornerstone of all health care, in this case the ability to preserve privacy and trust takes on special importance for two reasons. First is the recognition of the highly personalized nature of information about our mental and emotional states. It is, in many ways, the most personal information about any of us. Second is the stigma attached to mental illness. Children, adolescents, and families have suffered greatly as a result of the lingering myths and misconceptions about mental illness. We know that mental illnesses are treatable, but fear of incurring the label "mentally ill" prevents many from seeking treatment.

Despite the scientific progress in understanding mental illness, we have not seen equal progress in the reduction of the social stigma. In fact, we still hear stories about people denied employment, insurance, education, and other opportunities as a result of this pervasive stigma.

Our framework for addressing the privacy of mental health information should acknowledge the vulnerable position of individuals seeking mental health treatment, establish a firm commitment to sensitive and respectful consideration of the issues, and encourage the inclusion of those affected by decisions that will be rendered. Consumers, family members, legislators, mental health professionals, and others have wrestled with privacy and confidentiality concerns, yet consensus has been difficult to achieve. The Health Insurance Portability and Accountability Act (HIPAA) of 1996 has established timelines for making decisions about electronic health information transactions. Because of HIPAA and the public discussions of the decline of privacy in all aspects of life and its critical importance for mental health consumers, The Carter Center Mental Health Task Force decided to address the topic at its annual national symposium in 1997. The chapters that follow represent some of the work presented at that meeting and some additional efforts as well.

The breadth of the issues covered in this book reflects the complexity and diversity of interests in the privacy of mental health information. For example, it is not enough to explore the relevant technology without considering the impact on consumers and family members. Nor is it sufficient to explore the legal framework without attending to the special needs of children and adolescents. It is also difficult to discuss the sensitive nature of mental health information without acknowledging the similar stigma facing individuals with HIV and addictive disorders. These challenges require a comprehensive approach. A wealth of information has been gathered, and many diverse constituents have provided testimony on the subject. The intent of this book is to raise questions and concerns and to stimulate dialogue.

The greatest challenge is to craft a balance that provides individuals with thoughtful and reasonable protection while allowing for the appropriate release of information. Examples include information to payers, researchers, other providers, public health officials, oversight entities, and family members. In each case, our guiding question is, *Who needs what information for what purpose?* Historically, these decisions have been made with little uniformity and without enough input from consumers. Our approach must change so that consumers have the right to know what information is in their records, to whom that information will be released, and what they can do if they believe the records are inaccurate.

In response to HIPAA, decisions will be made in the near future and will be reevaluated as our health care system and technological capabilities continue to evolve. The more we do now to encourage the development of value-based decisions, the greater chance we have of developing laws and guidelines that address the needs of all parties who have a stake in the protection or the release of certain information. We must not permit the degree of difficulty involved to prevent us from taking a thoughtful, well-researched approach. We must keep at the core of our decision making a genuine concern for the individuals who will suffer if we fail to appreciate the complexity of this issue. Most important, we have a responsibility to ensure a consistent standard level of protection that individuals have a right to expect. Not only do we need to develop reasoned legislation, but we must improve our ability to articulate our standards, enforce our decisions, and establish guidelines for their violations. We can no longer be simply concerned about "someone else's" personal information. Growing awareness of the prevalence of mental illness and substance abuse issues in the United States reminds each of us that the information we are considering is never too far from our own.

When Jimmy Carter was president and established the President's Commission on Mental Health, I was pleased that we had the opportunity to propose many changes that would improve the lives of people with mental illness. Although the Mental Health Systems Act of 1980 was passed, the administration that followed us nullified it in 1981. Nevertheless, many of the ideas in the act became part of the mainstream of mental health services in the years that followed. As we prepare for the new millennium, we have another opportunity to help improve the quality of life of people with mental illness. By addressing the issues of privacy and confidentiality, we can serve the needs of individual consumers and the societal needs of all of us.

Rosalynn Carter
Chair
The Carter Center Mental Health Task Force

Foreword

Confidentiality of personal information has been a core ethical principle in all health care, incorporated into the ethics statements of most health professions. Yet, the need to safeguard sensitive health information disclosed during treatment continues to be a significant, even a growing, personal concern to many people seeking health services. Historically, medical record privacy has been a particular issue in the field of mental health, where this issue affects not only the relationship between doctor and patient but also the financing of services, the ways in which medical information is maintained by insurance companies, social matters such as housing and employment, and even the research on which we depend for new treatments of these disorders.

Why? The reality is that mental health issues—mental illnesses—are still the subject of considerable stigma. Inappropriately disclosed information about mental health issues may exact not only personal costs but also economic ones. Some years ago, it was common practice in both the federal and private sectors to "bundle" employee health records with personnel records. Consider the potentially damaging effect that a health record detailing mental health problems could have—and did have—on promotions, on continued employment or employment in the first place, and on personal and family reputations.

Although these very different kinds of records no longer are maintained in such close proximity, mental health information still can be used to an individual citizen's detriment. Several stories that have come to light amplify the continued need for real concern. An 18-year-old boy was denied health insurance coverage simply because he had received a few brief psychotherapy sessions 10 years earlier to help manage his grief following the death of a parent. A career employee with a successful work history in a field requiring discretion and privacy was dismissed when he was found to be using physician-prescribed medication to treat his diagnosed clinical depression.

To escape potential insurance difficulties and to free themselves from the fear of this sort of disclosure, a number of people have chosen to forgo insurance coverage payments and use cash or a check to pay for mental health services. Unfortunately, not everyone can afford to resolve the confidentiality conundrum in this way; moreover, they shouldn't be required to do so. Mental health issues should not have to be deep, dark, and hidden secrets that people must go to great lengths to hide from employers, insurers, and neighbors.

Increasingly, the same host of trust and confidentiality issues is reaching into the lives of countless other Americans who are experiencing or may someday experience different health problems. The excitement about new findings that link genetic information to predispositions for breast and colon cancer or the identification of genes that give rise to cystic fibrosis and Huntington's disease has been tempered with a cold dose of hard questions. Some are personal in nature, relating to individual choices in health care. Some affect a family, such as decisions about childbearing or whether to share knowledge of a gene-linked predisposition for illness with adolescent or young-adult children who might carry the same genetic pattern.

Another type of fallout from these new and exciting health findings, however, is more global in nature. What effect might this medical information have on employment and educational opportunities? Equally important, might this information be used to exclude individuals and their children from insurance coverage? The physical, economic, and personal tolls that the wrong answers to these questions would wreak is incalculable. However, it is increasingly evident that for equity, dignity, and individual security, basic confidentiality safeguards must be set in place for everyone.

Not surprisingly, the protection of confidentiality of health information increasingly is becoming an issue that extends beyond the mental health community and beyond the health community as a whole. Safeguarding confidential information is no longer a simple matter of locking the file cabinet in the doctor's office or in the personnel office. Most Americans feel very strongly that they, and not someone else, should have control over their personal information, whether it be their medical records or the conduct of their private lives. The question becomes one of how such protections are accomplished. After all, in this age of high-speed computers and telecommunications, information gets collected and used in so many unexpected ways. Some are overt, but other data collection methods are less obvious; we may not even be aware of them.

Just consider the electronic revolution and the effect the computer age is having on our lives. Some commercial web sites actually "learn" about your personal reading interests when you browse the site's contents, suggesting new sites to visit or choices to make based on that amassed knowledge. At some grocery stores, the scanner at the check-out counter not only totals your purchases but also keeps a record of your shopping habits. Shelves stocked with your favorite purchases and cents-off coupons reflect your culinary tastes. Each of these is a benign example of how technology is being used to catalog information about us. However, not all of the information catalogued is benign and not all of those with access to that information are necessarily using it in a harmless way.

A story in the newspaper detailed how pharmaceutical companies can use pharmacists' computerized prescription medicine records to target promotional advertising about specific new medications to specific physicians and their patients. That same computer record could help pharmacists keep track of potentially dangerous drug interactions from medicines prescribed for a single patient by more than one doctor. Whether both of these are appropriate uses of this information and whether the information should be privileged in one case and not in the other are not entirely clear. However, it is evident that data storage technologies and informatics have changed so rapidly that the laws and policies governing the protection of personal information have not been able to keep pace. It is equally evident that the gap needs to be spanned; we then must learn how to adjust our privacy policies to match future technological advances.

With the significant changes in how information is amassed and stored, everyone should be concerned with who has access to large databases containing medical information about individual citizens' illnesses, medications, and treatments. Certainly, many good reasons exist for gaining access to health care information contained in medical records: research, quality assurance, and public health protection, to name just a few. What is not as clear is precisely how much information is enough information for these purposes. Equally unclear is the range of individuals to whom even limited amounts of confidential health information should be disclosed. How should law enforcement personnel get health-related information about problems among the citizens they protect, and under what circumstances? Should schools and teachers be privy to confidential health information bearing on their students? How much private health information should be disclosed to family members who are acting as caregivers? Are the answers to these questions the same or different for physical illnesses, mental health illnesses, and substance abuse problems? Answers to these questions are difficult at best. Physicians who are asked to answer such questions often face complex moral and ethical decisions. What is clear, however, is that great care must be taken to circumscribe what information is made available, to whom it is made available, and to what purpose it is being put, as the decision could have profound human effects.

I support my husband, Vice President Al Gore's proposal of an Electronic Bill of Rights for this electronic age that would embody four central principles: 1) the right to choose whether your personal information is disclosed; 2) the right to know how, when, and how much of that information is being used; 3) the right to see the information yourself; and 4) the right to know whether it is accurate and to correct it if it is not.

Unfortunately, today, the laws are not always clear; what is acceptable in one state may not be acceptable in another. We have an opportunity to do something about this by setting basic national standards. The 1996 Kennedy-Kassebaum health care bill required the U.S. Department of Health and Human Services to recommend federal legislation to this end. The Department did just that by addressing confidentiality issues within the context of a Consumer Bill of Rights and Responsibilities that ensures that the health care system is both fair and responsive to consumer needs. That document is being implemented across the federal government. Among its broad range of interrelated consumer rights, the Consumer Bill of Rights and Responsibilities specifies that health care consumers have the right to communicate with their health care providers in confidence; their individually identifiable health care information shall remain confidential. Moreover, it states that consumers have the right to receive accurate, easily understood information about their own health care, their health plan, and their health care professionals and facilities. If inaccuracies exist in a consumer's health record, the individual may request corrections. Perhaps most important, the document posits that consumers have the right to considerate, respectful care from all members of the health care industry, at all times, and under all circumstances; they cannot be discriminated against in marketing, enrollment practices, or service delivery.

Corollary to these and other consumer rights are a number of consumer responsibilities that emphasize the need for individuals to take responsibility for their health-related habits, that encourage provision of relevant information related to treatment they may require, and, importantly, that urge clear two-way communication between consumers and the health care system.

These activities at the federal level, although an important part of the process of protecting confidentiality, are but one part of a larger process that must take place nationwide. We need to pay attention to these issues in public policy, in academic training, in community programming, and in business practices so that individual clinicians can focus more appropriately on providing high-quality mental health and other health care services. At the same time, we must be able to reassure the American people that their health information is safeguarded, allowing people to clear a key barrier to needed diagnostic and treatment services.

The discussions at The Carter Center Symposium in 1997 and the creative and analytic thinking contained in this book delineate the range of issues that must be addressed if we are to ensure that medical confidentiality issues are considered and respected not only in mental health but also in all health care fields. They also pose a challenge, in this age of instant information and communications technology, to policy makers and program leaders, to those in business and research, and to those in technology and informatics to collaborate in the development and implementation of a nationwide solution to the crisis in health care confidentiality that will endure long into the 21st century.

Tipper Gore

Acknowledgments

Because much of this book originated in the planning of the Thirteenth Annual Rosalynn Carter Symposium on Mental Health Policy held at The Carter Center in Atlanta, Georgia, in 1997, it is important to acknowledge the contributions of those who helped to plan that meeting. Following the agreement between The Carter Center and The Center for Mental Health Services to collaborate on the planning of the symposium, a planning committee was formed in early 1997 to discuss alternative approaches to the complex topic of privacy and confidentiality, identify key issues, and develop a list of potential contributors (authors, speakers, and panelists). The editors of this book co-chaired the two meetings of the committee and were ably assisted by Judy Fitzgerald, M.S.W., of The Carter Center Mental Health Program and staff members of The Center for Mental Health Services, which included Catherine Acuff, Ph.D.; Seth Hassett, M.S.W.; Norma Hatot, Captain of the U.S. Public Health Service; and Judith Katz-Leavy, M.Ed. Financial support for the work of the planning committee and the symposium itself was provided by The Center for Mental Health Services of the Substance Abuse and Mental Health Services Administration, U.S. Department of Health and Human Services, The John D. and Catherine T. MacArthur Foundation, The Robert Wood Johnson Foundation, and WXIA-TV, 11 Alive Gannett Communities Fund.

The knowledge, experience, and hard work of the following members of the planning committee are gratefully acknowledged: Robert Bernstein, Ph.D., Executive Director of the Bazelon Center for Mental Health Law; Thomas E. Bryant, M.D., J.D., The Carter Center Mental Health Task Force, and Chairman, Non-Profit Management Associates, Inc.; Augusta Gross, Ph.D., psychologist in private practice and health consultant to the office of Mrs. Tipper Gore; Barbara Guthrie, R.N., Ph.D., the School of Nursing at the University of Michigan; Richard Harding, M.D., psychiatrist in private practice and a member of the National Committee on Vital and Health Statistics; Skila Harris, former chief of staff to Mrs. Tipper Gore; Jo Hill, Oklahoma Mental Health Consumer Council; Kimberly Hoagwood, Ph.D., National Institute of Mental Health; Marylin Levitt, D.S.W., health consultant to the office of Mrs. Tipper

Gore; Elisabeth Rukeyser, mental health advocate and former member, National Advisory Mental Health Council, The Center for Mental Health Services; Beth Stroul, M.Ed., consultant on children's mental health services; and Laura Van Tosh, consumer advocate with experience in public and private health care sectors.

We wish to offer special thanks to the authors of the chapters in this book for their hard work and scholarship and also for their patience and perseverance as we went back to them on more than one occasion to ask questions, seek clarification, and otherwise attend to many editorial details. In addition to the authors, another group of people provided critical commentaries at the symposium on the six papers commissioned at that time. As such, they helped the authors to review and refine their original manuscripts, and we thus acknowledge the commentaries provided by Richard Harding, M.D.; Ray Patterson, M.D.; Valerie Burrell-Muhammad; Don Richardson, Ph.D.; Steven Sharfstein, M.D., M.P.A.; and Darby Penney.

Our work as editors was greatly facilitated by the diligent and competent assistance of Judy Fitzgerald at The Carter Center and Judith Katz-Leavy and Norma Hatot of The Center for Mental Health Services. Their assistance with the review of manuscripts, organization of the chapters, administration of contracts, and critical thinking helped immeasurably. Their contributions are deeply appreciated.

Mention must also be made of the staff at The Carter Center, whose help with proofreading, typing, communications, and correspondence enabled the completion of the book. Many thanks go to Lei Ellingson, M.P.P., current assistant director of The Carter Center Mental Health Program; again to Judy Fitzgerald for her continuing above-and-beyond efforts since resigning as the assistant director; Lynne Randolph, administrative assistant; and Valerie Thompson, secretary.

Finally, we acknowledge with respect and admiration the leadership of Rosalynn Carter, without whom the symposium, the book, and so much else of value to people with mental illness would not have occurred. We also express our thanks to Tipper Gore for her contributions to the symposium and the book and for her efforts to advance the mental health agenda.

In loving memory of my parents
J.J.G.

To my mother, Sally Arons
B.S.A.

Privacy and Confidentiality in Mental Health Care

1

Introduction

John J. Gates and Bernard S. Arons

Protecting privacy and confidentiality has been of great importance to people with mental illness because of the stigma and discrimination that they have experienced. Because of pervasive ignorance and misunderstanding about mental illness, erroneous stereotypes and myths have persisted throughout the 20th century. Although research (Gollub & Hyman, 1996; Gorman & Papp, 1994) on the structure and functioning of the brain and advances in treatments have helped to begin to change public attitudes, many of the stereotypes and myths continue. Widespread beliefs that most people with mental illness are dangerous, undependable, untreatable, and somehow responsible for their problems are conveyed to those with mental illness, compounding their emotional and mental difficulties with feelings of shame and embarrassment. One result is that many individuals suffer in silence and isolation, neither discussing their difficulties with family and friends nor seeking the care and treatment that they need, fearing that to do so would reveal their "shameful" secret. They fear not only this sense of being marked or stigmatized but also the practical consequences of what others might do to them if it were known that they have a mental illness. These consequences include people being denied jobs for which they are qualified, not receiving promotions that their work performance justifies, not securing a loan or line of credit that financial facts would ordinarily warrant, and being denied an insurance policy or being offered one with much higher premiums than the standard (National Organization on Disabilities/Louis Harris & Associates, 1998; Reich, 1998). Although the Americans with Disabilities Act (ADA) of 1990 (PL 101-336) has made many of these practices illegal, evidence suggests that they persist (Spayd, 1998). Stigma and discrimination are real, hence the continuing concern to protect privacy and confidentiality.

Changes in the delivery and financing of health care in the United States have heightened concern about privacy and confidentiality. The evolution of managed care has expanded third-party presence in the consumer–provider (patient, client) relationship. The accompanying "corporatization" of health care delivery (i.e., the migration of hundreds of thousands of diverse health care providers from their private offices to corporate groups, networks, and systems) has affected the relationships of trust and personal confidence between patients and their caregivers that were the norm throughout most of the 20th century—indeed, perhaps since the time of Hippocrates more than 2,000 years ago (Feldman, Novack, & Gracely, 1998; Simon et al., 1999). The growth of the health care corporations has occurred in tandem with the growth of large databases of health care information stored and transmitted electronically, increasingly across state boundaries. Access to this sensitive information by a seemingly larger and larger number of entities (health care providers, payers, utilization reviewers, researchers, employers, public health professionals, fraud investigators, claims processors, administrative staff, law enforcement agents, and court officials) has caused alarm about the potential misuse of the information by both authorized and unauthorized users.

As a result of the developments mentioned previously, there has been renewed interest in developing legislation and policy that will guide information management practices in the future. Bills have been introduced in the Congress and in many state legislatures, and discussions of the issues have proliferated in academia; in corporate board rooms (health maintenance organizations, managed care companies, insurance companies, corporations whose health benefit plans pay for much health care); and among associations of consumers, family members, and providers (e.g., physicians, nurses, psychologists, social workers). It has been difficult to achieve consensus because the issues are complex and involve a fundamental question of the right of the individual to personal privacy and the needs of society to place limitations on that right.

This book explores the issue of the protection of privacy and the confidentiality of health care information from a number of perspectives. The special perspectives of consumers and family members are developed in Chapters 2 (Campbell) and 3 (Lefley), respectively, and Chapter 4 (Melton) discusses the special issues regarding the privacy and confidentiality of children and adolescents. Clinical, legal, and technological issues are identified and explored in Chapters 5 (Goin), 6 (Petrila), and 7 (Gellman), respectively. Chapters 8 (Barret) and 9 (Samuels), which discuss HIV/AIDS and substance abuse issues, respectively, were added because people who experience these disorders also experience stigma and discrimination when information regarding their illness is misused. Chapter 10 (Gates & Fitzgerald) brings focus to the fundamental importance of personal privacy and the public good that comes from both its protection and its limits and also recommends one approach to balance the two. The opinions expressed are strictly those of the author(s) of each chapter. The appendix at the end of the book (Petrila) provides a useful and succinct summary of state mental health laws.

Both health care practices and information management practices will continue to change, enabled by advances in medical technology and information-processing technology, simultaneously improving and threatening our ability to protect privacy and confidentiality and challenging existing laws and policies. It is likely that the laws and policies will need to be reviewed and revised from time to time. It is hoped that the issues and perspectives discussed in this book will be useful to all those interested in developing practices that benefit the needs of individual consumers and of society as a whole.

REFERENCES

Americans with Disabilities Act (ADA) of 1990, PL 101-336, 42 U.S.C. §§ 12101 *et seq.*

Feldman, D., Novack, D., & Gracely, E. (1998). Effects of managed care on physician–patient relationships, quality of care, and the ethical practice of medicine: A physician survey. *Archive of Internal Medicine, 158*(15), 1626–1632.

Gollub, R.L., & Hyman, S.E. (1996). Recent advances in neuroscience relevant to psychiatry [Foreword to Section III]. In L.J. Dickstein, M.B. Riba, & J.M. Oldham (Eds.), *Review of psychiatry* (Vol. 15, pp. 275–279). Washington, DC: American Psychiatric Press.

Gorman, J.M., & Papp, L.A. (1994). Biological markers [Foreword to Section II]. In J.M. Oldham & M.B. Riba (Eds.), *Review of psychiatry* (Vol. 13, pp. 129–132). Washington, DC: American Psychiatric Press.

National Organization on Disabilities/Louis Harris & Associates. (1998). Closing the gaps: 1998. Results from an N.O.D./Harris survey of Americans with disabilities. *Disability Agenda, 1*(2).

Reich, A. (1998). Closing the gaps: A call for community action. *Disability Agenda, 1*(2), 1–2.

Simon, S., Pan, R., Sullivan, A., Clarke-Chiarelli, N., Connelly, M., Peters, A., Singer, J., Inui, T., & Block, S. (1999). Views of managed care: A survey of students, residents, faculty, and deans at medical schools in the United States. *New England Journal of Medicine, 340*(12), 928–936.

Spayd, L. (1998, July 22). Poll finds harsh life for disabled. *The Washington Post,* p. A1.

2

Consumers' Perspective of Confidentiality and Health Records

Jean Campbell

The United States has been propelled irretrievably into an era of computers and electronic networks. With this technology has come the ability and the desire to employ it in the health care field by developing databases of medical records. Electronic linkage of medical records promises improved care, both at the system level and at the individual level of service utilization. However, consumers worry that their information could be misused by both authorized and unauthorized users. Within the general debate regarding privacy and confidentiality of health records, this chapter analyzes the demands of health consumers to control the use of their own health data within health management information systems.

THE DILEMMA

The development and implementation of managed health care plans depend on information about individuals in order to determine who should be enrolled, to set rates, to determine quality and effectiveness of services, and to engage in prior and concurrent review. Personal health data have become a refined commodity that has considerable worth in the health care marketplace. Most important, the capacity to transmit patient-specific information within the network of providers greatly benefits consumers. Access to computerized information can integrate individual care rather than keep each medical episode a discrete, unrelated event (Petrila, 1996). For example, the name of a person's psychiatrist or medication records could be available instantly to doctors in a psychiatric emergency room, even though the individual who is being evaluated might not be able to provide this information. Also, the repeated collection of a person's medical history could be eliminated, saving the staff and the consumer much time and effort.

However, people care deeply about their medical information. It is personal. The risks of exposure of medical records that can profoundly change people's lives are multiplying. With increasing frequency, the public reads or hears of cases in which individuals have lost insurance, jobs, and housing or have been subjected to public humiliation because of something in their medical records. "Whether HIV, cancer, diabetes, or some other health problem, companies are using the information to decide who gets hired, fired, and promoted" (Stanley & Palosky, 1997d). The following incidents are just a few examples taken from an in-depth series of articles on medical privacy published in *The Tampa Tribune* (Palosky & Stanley, 1997a, 1997c; Stanley & Palosky, 1997d):

- A Tampa woman never expected anyone to learn about her sessions with a therapist, but when she got hurt in a car accident and sued, defense lawyers claimed that her problems were mental, not physical. At the trial, an attorney read to the jury from the therapist's notes the details of her past emotional problems. "I looked like a crazy person, and I lost the case," reported the woman.
- In California, a state agency denied a man a job in part because he had been treated for depression.
- When Rep. Nydia Velaquez (D-NY) first ran for Congress in 1992, the *New York Post* published details about her past suicide attempt. She won the election and later sued her hospital for failing to protect her records.
- The names of 4,000 people on a Florida state–created list of AIDS patients were copied from a state computer and mailed to newspapers.

Inadvertent breaches of confidentiality, health data searches by law enforcement agencies, and the myriad of data-merging activities that are taking place have created a chilling effect on people who seek medical help. Stigmatized populations, such as people with mental illness, HIV/AIDS, or alcohol and substance abuse problems, are the most vulnerable to violations of health privacy because the practical consequences of being identified are extreme.

In general, medical privacy issues of a person who has bipolar disorder do not differ substantially from those of someone who is HIV positive. Not only have such people been victimized by their disease, but they also have been forced to confront attendant prejudice, discrimination, and public fear. Medical privacy, therefore, looms over their everyday lives and must be addressed within the critical context of civil liberties.

ACCESS TO DATA

It was not long ago that transmission of a medical record meant that the file was put into a pneumatic tube and sucked away to another part of the hospital. Clinicians' handwritten progress notes, which once were kept in manila folders in locked file cabinets, are giving way to vast electronic warehouses that store, integrate, and link data. The growth of a national health data infrastructure coupled with technological advances in electronic data management provide health care systems with the capacity both horizontally and vertically to integrate, synthesize, and use health information with few restraints (Gostin, Lazzarini, Neslund, & Osterholm, 1996). Most of this is being accomplished without the knowledge or permission of health care recipients (Campbell, 1997b).

Privacy and confidentiality for the individual consumer implies that access to personal health data and clinical records is limited by informed consent, the law, medical ethics, and state and national policies that protect the consumer, the consumer's family, and the provider agencies that collect and manage data and clinical records. However, as the power of information systems grows, ethical, financial, and technological dilemmas emerge to challenge such protections. Most people do not realize who sees their medical data. Harvard law professor Arthur Miller said, "It's like the genie springing out of the bottle, going anywhere on the planet for any purpose whatsoever" (Stanley & Palosky, 1997a). Self-insured employers often review medical information such as doctors' bills and prescription records to track their health plan's expenses. Health maintenance organizations often require detailed data about patients before they approve treatment. In some states, regulators collect social security numbers (SSNs) and other data about every person who enters a hospital or an alcohol/drug treatment center.

Furthermore, with the emphasis on patient tracking and controlling health costs through outcome-based decision making, the potential for misuse of health data in services research has increased enormously. Researchers have liberal access to records, in-

cluding those of people with stigmatizing conditions. The trend toward increasingly rigorous evaluation of services through research
in the community and in institutions and the expanding influence
of consumers, family members, and advocates in the research and
data collection arena have clouded traditional protections and compromised boundaries of taken-for-granted ethical authority and protocol (Campbell & Estroff, 1995). Most attention in the field has
been focused on ethical dilemmas in neurobiological research—
especially experimental psychotropic drug research (Burd, 1995;
Weisburd, 1994)—leaving protocols that protect data subjects in a
regulatory gray zone. The important ethical questions that behavioral health providers and services researchers now face in their investigations have seldom been addressed, and the data community
has yet to achieve consensus about standards and policy recommendations (Campbell, 1996b).

As the federal government initiates national medical privacy
standards that can accommodate the new technologies, it is important to recognize that promises of better services are not persuasive
either for the general public or for vulnerable populations. In fact,
the causation among linkage of records, outcomes studies, and
quality of services has yet to be proved in the scientific community.

Public attitudes reflect overwhelming support for more controls regarding medical privacy. The 1993 Equifax Harris Consumer
Privacy Survey (Electronic Privacy Information Center [EPIC],
1999) found that 75% of people in the United States worry that
medical information from a computerized national health information system will be used for many nonhealth reasons, and 38% are
very concerned. Although most said that it was important that individuals have the legal right to obtain a copy of their own medical
record, 85% believed that protecting the confidentiality of medical
records is "absolutely essential" or "very important" in health care
reform; 56% favored new comprehensive legislation to protect the
privacy of medical records, and 64% did not want medical researchers to use their records for studies—even if the individual is
never identified—unless researchers first get the individual's consent. Of those surveyed, 96% supported federal legislation that
would designate all personal medical information as "sensitive"
and impose penalties for unauthorized disclosure. The "Live and
Let Live" American Civil Liberties Union (ACLU) poll in 1994 also
found that 75% of those surveyed are concerned a "great deal" or a
"fair amount" about insurance companies' putting medical information about them into a computer information bank to which
others have access (EPIC, 1999). Similarly, a 1996 CNN poll found

that 87% of Americans believed that patients should be asked permission every time any information about them is used (EPIC, 1999).

It is clear that an improperly thought out and implemented data system can result in invasion of privacy, personal surveillance, abridgment of constitutional rights, inappropriate monitoring and control of individuals, and access to personal data for private profit or criminal use. Besides anxiety about information leaks, most people have a natural reluctance to be tracked and monitored in the most personal aspects of their lives. By expanding the scope and capacity of electronic information systems, personal autonomy is eroded even when records can be secured. Both of these types of privacy concerns produce adverse medical and public health consequences. People do not tell the whole story to doctors when they fear that they or their friends and relatives will be harmed as a result of leaks in the health information system or that "Big Brother" is watching. It is the expectation of privacy that leads to trust in the doctor–patient relationship. Without the confidence that a physician will hold private the most intimate facts of a person's life, patients do not reveal themselves. Consequently, treatment can be hindered or delayed. In testimony to the National Committee on Vital and Health Statistics (NCVHS), George Flores, M.D. (1997), a public health professional, stated,

> Public health holds an unique position in access to and the need to work with sensitive client information. In order to be able to make contact with persons having contagious conditions and to have the cooperation and trust of their medical providers, the door to public health must be open to all categories of individuals, including those who may be disadvantaged by disclosure of their identity. For the door to be open, there must be public confidence in the privacy and security of medical information. This holds true for medical as well as mental health clients, their medical records, and, in many cases, their identities.

Mental health consumers share similar concerns regarding medical health privacy with those who have illegally immigrated to the United States. Some people with mental illness choose to stay away from mental health services because they also fear that an encounter would put themselves, a family member, or a friend in a threatening position. They could potentially be stigmatized and the information used against them to deny work, custody of children, or even freedom. However, not seeking services could cause an exacerbation in symptoms for people with mental illness, putting themselves and others at risk. The point is that lack of privacy assurances in health data collection has been shown to adversely affect help-seeking behaviors and, subsequently, precipitate public health problems.

Protections and issues of control of access to medical records are not rigorously evaluated in terms of their impact on health consumers, and consumers' voices often are not represented when standards are being developed. Health privacy ultimately is a struggle over control of health records and is more related to issues of informed consent and ownership of records than to security. What is ironic is that security concerns and recommended protocols for electronic health records restrict consumers' access to their own records but do little to control the use of the records in management information systems. In fact, most efforts to develop medical privacy standards in the United States proceed from the assumption that access by third parties, including provider networks, billing companies, law enforcement, and researchers, is necessary, and most protections being drafted accommodate demands for data linkage and transmission.

Beyond issues of security and controlled access to medical records, other struggles are being waged under the banner of medical privacy. Obviously, ideas and perspectives are powerful tools of both social change and control, especially when they are coupled with data. The production of medical information has had considerable influence on determining health policies related to treatment and cost. The corporate and public behavioral health systems that manage medical records may have vested interests in restricting information that reflects negatively on their organizations. Such data have the potential to validate criticism of health service delivery systems. Where data often serve to justify the status quo, issues of data access and control provide fertile ground for a discussion of values and the attitudes and behaviors of professionals in executing data collection protocols and distributing results of performance-based studies (Campbell & Estroff, 1995; Petrila, 1996; Wedding, Topolski, & McGaha, 1995).

If the sense of what is right is equivocal and dialogue is submerged in taken-for-granted practices, then who or what policy mechanisms are capable of defining ethical codes or developing surveillance systems to monitor discrete behaviors within the data collection process? With privatization of health care has come the weakening of the oversight and regulatory roles of the federal government. Furthermore, data conflicts involve complex reciprocal social and personal relationships. How are choices negotiated between individual gain and the greater good, or individual good and the greater gain? Do the ends now justify the means as efforts to manage by outcomes suggest? Following orders of superiors and sometimes even engaging in unethical behaviors are rewarded in health care entrepreneurialism, whereas whistle blowing or making an individual choice to break an unjust law spells corporate death.

History teaches that principles of "The Good" or "The Right" are not necessarily consensual but rather political. They flow from the top down through the state and bureaucratic structures, where they are codified in law, contract language, or become part of a set of informal protocols. However, what may be most compelling in prescribing standards of behavior and practice is the weight of aggregated private decision making of middle-level managers on public and corporate policies. Private fears and desires for gain or recognition become a latent infrastructure, invisible to the system at the organizational level but manifest to individual participants as "the rules of the game." Protecting medical privacy becomes a colluded process that is situational and self-justifying. Protections and protocols, while grounded in custom and organizational history, are actually reflective of personal acts expressed as organizational will (Campbell, 1997a).

Mandating privacy protocols and technologies packed with security features is useless if people do not aggressively use these strategies. Although rules and regulations can provide pressure to control abuse, compliance inextricably will be subverted without the development of a profound respect by all constituencies for the value and worth of individual consumers. One need only to look at the violations of privacy and confidentiality that occur daily from the cavalier way that people handle and transmit data within low-tech systems to understand the nature and magnitude of the problem within electronic data infrastructures. The nature of privacy compliance problems are illustrated in the following account:

> While working at a state department of mental health, I encountered considerable resistance when I attempted to institute privacy protections around the use of a facsimile machine that received consumer-specific information. As I walked through the central offices, I often found lists of the names of patients at the state hospital lying in the fax machine or rolled up on the floor. I was the only one who seemed to notice or to care. When I recommended that a fax machine dedicated to receiving such information be put in a locked room or that client-specific information not be transmitted by fax, the only accommodation made was to place a portable room divider around one side of the machine.
>
> Later, at a research institution where I was subsequently employed, I observed that surveys of mental health consumers with respondent names on the cover sheets were routinely left in plain sight in an un-

locked room. Again, I was the only one who seemed to notice or to care. I reminded people that informed consent of consumers to participate in the survey was a contract between the respondents and the researchers who promised that the surveys would be kept in a locked file. Eventually the door was locked, but when electrical repairs to the room were made, a desk from that room with a red file labeled "Confidential Client Information" sat on the desktop in the hallway until I finally removed the file and took it to my supervisor. (J. Campbell, personal observation, 1997)

From such experiences, one can begin to recognize that many people do not connect mental health data with individuals. By carelessly handling someone's mental health record, people fail to realize that they are treating that person in a disrespectful, dehumanizing manner. Protection of privacy and confidentiality of mental health data becomes a collection of rules and protocols that people begrudgingly follow; they are not necessarily vigilant. Perhaps it is the stigmatized role of consumers and the "them and us" mentality of professionals that sustain a general lack of genuine concern within the culture of mental health services research.

The inherent tension around who should have access to health data and issues of confidentiality of health records have vast implications for the production and distribution of health information, but data collection policies and protocols also have an impact on the development of the cultural reference points that underlie every aspect of the personal and social relationships between professionals and consumers in the data collection, storage, and utilization process. Ultimately, the social relationships of health data management have the potential to alter the symbolic processes by which a consumer's reality is produced, maintained, repaired, and transformed. For this reason alone, the rights of consumers should be put first.

CONSUMERISM VERSUS PATERNALISM

The growing tide of health consumerism is one of the most compelling forces in carving out a role for mental health consumers in the production, storage, and use of their health data. It is based on the assumption that people who seek health services are customers just as are people who seek other types of services. The doctor is perceived to be the purveyor of a service, and the patient is viewed as the buyer. The consumer listens to the thoughts of the provider but ultimately makes his or her own decisions. *Consumerism* implies that values derived from principles of good medical care must be interpreted and operationalized through reference to the patient's personal health care values and desires (Beisecker & Beisecker, 1993).

Although consumerism has periodically emerged as a force in American society, its application in health care draws its roots from two marketplace trends: consumer rights protections, with its concerns regarding manufacturing and product safety, and total quality management, with its focus on customer satisfaction. The former is grounded in individuals' profound distrust of the actions and motives of providers of products and services; the latter promotes collaboration between provider and consumer and seeks to answer such questions as, "What do customers prefer?" It is important to recognize that both trends emphasize the need for information that accommodates consumer rights and interests.

Contrast this vision of consumerism with the fear, anger, and sadness often conveyed when people speak about violations to the privacy and confidentiality of their own health records. These experiences stand as a robust critique of management information systems and consumer rights and protections in health services research. It is not surprising that managers and scientists have been unable to cope with growing demands for changes in the data management process, particularly those that come from people with stigmatizing conditions and from their families. Paternalism, not consumerism, would appear to remain the reigning ethos in the management of health information. The American Psychiatric Association has repeatedly lobbied Congress when health data access and confidentiality legislation was being considered to prevent a person's access to his or her personal psychiatric records. Such restrictions on access have been legislated by many states and are supported in *Confidentiality of Individually-Identifiable Health Information: Recommendations of the Secretary of Health and Human Services, pursuant to section 264 of the Health Insurance Portability and Accountability Act of 1996* (U.S. Department of Health and Human Services [DHHS], 1997). Mental health professionals fear that giving broad access rights to mental health consumers may pose a danger to an individual's psychological health. As with science in general, psychiatric research is bound by the past and inscribed with power, bias, and stereotypy. Reform in research methods, protocols, and human subjects' protections historically has been based on the assumption that "the expert knows best" about the operating principles of research. Furthermore, scientists believe that they know the values and preferences of their subjects, that they are disinterested and objective without biases of their own, and that they can choose for their subjects what the subjects would choose for themselves if they had the same knowledge. This seduction by authority inevitably influences future behavior to mimic current practices and thus leads to the creation of data protocols and protections without knowledge of how consumers would address these issues.

REIFICATION OF SYSTEM VALUES

One of the most disturbing claims to override consumers' rights to confidentiality is the need for outcome studies. Such studies not only may involve the use of psychiatric records without consent but also may require that service recipients fill out intrusive questionnaires as a condition of their treatment. Consumers question the value of this type of research and ask whether system values—in this instance, the potential for lower costs and more effective treatment modalities—trump the value of respect for individual autonomy. In response to Nazi atrocities in the conduct of human experimentation, the Nuremberg Code proclaimed as its first principle that "the voluntary consent of the human subject is absolutely essential" (Katz, 1972, p. 305). One of the most well-respected historical documents concerning the use of human subjects in medical research, it requires that "the person . . . should be able to exercise free choice without intervention of any element of force . . . or coercion" (p. 305). Scientists who justify the widespread use of outcome studies are really amending this fundamental premise of patient consent for research by advancing public goals. If outcome studies and other services' research activities were included under human subjects' protections, then individual benefit—not public benefit— would have to be weighed by the consumer against potential risks of data collection in an informed consent protocol.

Fearing loss of enrollees, contracts, and public scrutiny, administrators of public and private health delivery systems are claiming proprietary rights of data ownership to control access to information (Petersen, 1995). Often, when public agencies and private companies pay for data collection, they demand the right to prohibit the review or publication of health service system information without their permission. State mental health authorities may impose similar limitations on researchers as to the presentation, publication, or review of data, and access to services research is denied to the public when results are potentially unfavorable. In these ways, academic freedom and the public's right to know—even when federal and state money is used—are silently being undermined by system-centered concerns regarding disclosure of information.

Finally, there is an eagerness by those in politics to reveal personal health information to gain advantage, and instances in which privacy protections have been put aside in the service of public policy are not new. This complicates the role of government as the protector of medical privacy. Consider the case of Daniel Ellsberg (Hayden, 1988; Robitscher, 1981; *World Book Year Book,* 1974; Zinn, 1990). The first public act in the Watergate cover-up was not the break-in at the Watergate Hotel, but a break-in 9 months earlier for psychiatric information to discredit Ellsberg, who had turned against the Vietnam War. Ellsberg had copied volumes of secret Defense Department papers and made them available to *The New York Times* while he was working for the Rand Corporation as a government consultant. He said that he released the information because the American people had a right to know about the actions of their government. The Supreme Court upheld the right of newspapers to print the material, ruling that the government's attempt to suppress publication was "prior restraint of freedom of the press" and, therefore, unconstitutional. However, Ellsberg was still indicted for espionage, theft, and conspiracy. Ultimately, the case was dismissed after 89 days because of a number of violations of procedure, including the illegal break-in at the office of Ellsberg's psychiatrist. The judge labeled such behavior as "improper government conduct, shielded so long from public view" that offended "a sense of justice" (*World Book Year Book,* 1974, p. 307).

Proposed legislation might well allow federal and state agencies the very type of access that once was gained only through covert activities. It has been reported that recommendations by the Clinton administration regarding medical privacy would permit health care providers and those who pay for such services to be explicitly permitted to disclose health information without authorization when the records are sought by federal or state investigators. Furthermore, as part of the Brady Handgun Violence Prevention Act (1993), a national computerized background check will include access to psychiatric hospital records to prevent people who have been hospitalized from purchasing handguns (Applebaum & Monahan, 1994).

Because vested interests, bureaucracies, and corporate entities have greater opportunities to affect health privacy policies than do individuals or public advocacy groups (Breitenstein & Nagel, 1997; Nagel, 1998), government agencies are inhibited from rigorously promoting standards and penalties that give priority to individuals to determine appropriate access and use of medical information. The institutions that control information define by default or feel empowered to determine appropriate use and to minimize the concerns of private citizens. Consequently, administrators strive for as much access to information as possible, and data warehousing and merging technologies rapidly develop to meet the demand. There is little vision or incentive to develop systems that facilitate broad and meaningful consumer control of health records. Rather, services research designs and electronic health information architecture are considered unable to accommodate consumer demands. The creation of a national review body to provide oversight of medical records privacy and respond to health consumer concerns was rejected by the National Committee on Vital and Health Statistics in its recommendations to the Secretary of the DHHS because "no clear and practical solutions" (NCVHS, 1997, p. 26) are offered as rationale, with little interrogation of the underlying assumptions for this position or alternatives sought.

PUTTING THE RIGHTS OF CONSUMERS FIRST

It is evident that health consumers prioritize their needs for control over their personal health records above any needs promulgated by the government, researchers, or private industry. However, when the dialogue is shifted away from individual consumers to discussions of people at the system level, calls for a delicate balancing act between giving organizations what they need to know and individual rights repeatedly surface (Gates, 1998; U.S. DHHS, 1997). The argument is that widespread abuse can be controlled and health privacy can be regulated. When used and secured properly, electronic medical records can help patients and serve the public benefit. Therefore, privacy rights should never be absolute, and policy makers should chart a middle ground between those who want unfettered access and those who want stricter safeguards to ensure individual control over any use of one's medical record. The problem is that the concerns and solutions of health consumers as reflected in the national polls, and surveys have not adequately weighed in on the debate. Any abstract balance that is championed is strictly in the eyes of those at the table.

Rather than a shared reality based on market relations, data collection represents two quite separate worlds, and the meanings of one are significantly different from the other. Separated by role and function from the consumer, both public agencies and private corporations construct a rationale that tends to be antagonistic to individual rights to medical privacy.

What emerges when balancing the rights of health consumers with the demand for more personal medical data to be stored and moved electronically is a turf war over controlling human beings in a landscape that includes an entire array of options and widely divergent goals and definitions of fair information practices. The same policies appear as positive from one perspective, negative from another. When defining the cost and feasibility of protections and rights, most stakeholders look at the way it affects the system, whereas the individual consumer will ask, "What does it do to my life?"

For example, researchers will often protest when issues regarding privacy and confidentiality create barriers to their research but may reverse their opinions when health privacy protections affect them directly as a health consumer. Consider the following anecdote:

> As a member of a group reviewing grant applications, I found that my persistent concerns regarding the human subjects' protections were met with irritation. However, when we discussed a proposal for a data warehouse that would have direct impact on the medical records of some of the reviewers themselves, the mood changed dramatically. (J. Campbell, personal observation, April 1996)

In this case, the capacity to track people with behavioral health care problems was considered more important to the researcher than the individual rights of "those people" until the issue was made personal.

Because people judge benefit and harm of medical information systems by the impact on the quality of their individual lives, it is the individual perspective that needs to be at the core of the debate on medical privacy. However, individual concerns are often marginalized to infrequent opportunities for input at public hearings or shuffled aside in misdirected letters or telephone calls that go nowhere.

WHOSE DATA ARE THEY ANYWAY?

To empower individual health consumers to reposition their concerns within the center of power, it is necessary to introduce to the policy-making process the concept of consumer ownership of medical records (Campbell, 1996b). Rather than being regarded as health partners, consumers feel that that their mental health experiences are really viewed as raw data that can be mined, processed, and sold by entrepreneurs, corporations, and academia without much care for the welfare of the individual (Campbell, 1996b). In fact, it is rare that consumers are reimbursed for the burden of answering hours of questions for quality management or outcomes research, and they do not share in the profits—whether financial or professional. The situation is akin to a form of colonialism. Consumers are treated more like a captive population whose insights and practices are considered the property of the developer than a market exchange relationship of customer and service provider.

In the novel *The Deus Machine,* Ovellette (1993) created a near-future scenario of the first serious attempts to integrate the government's computer networks and the reaction from groups concerned with protecting the individual's rights to privacy. That fictional struggle was resolved through legislation that declared that personal data were extensions of "person" as defined in the Fourth Amendment to the Bill of Rights. Therefore, health data were protected against search and seizure, and officials were required to obtain a search warrant before linking and integrating data. The author asked the reader to think of health care data as an individual's personal effects, as something unique with private meaning and value, rather than as a saleable commodity belonging to a corporate or governmental agency. In the struggle over control of individual medical records, mental health consumers are beginning to advance proprietary arguments (Campbell, 1996b). Although there is as yet little case law to support such claims to data ownership, consumers are engaging the legal system as a means to protect and control the use of private health data, to gain access to and direct the collection of system-level information, and to share in the profits from data production and use. Most important, they seek a forum to become leaders in the development of health information system protocols and protections to accomplish these objectives.

PAVING THE WAY OR PROTECTING THE INDIVIDUAL?

When the Health Insurance Portability and Accountability Act (HIPAA) of 1996 (PL 104-191) created portability and more coverage for preexisting conditions, it added at the last moment a provision to facilitate the computerization of medical records in national databases run by the government and private corporations. Congress, with the advice of the NCVHS, directed the Secretary of the DHHS to make "detailed recommendations on standards with respect to the privacy of individually identifiable health information" in HIPAA, section 264(a). In making those recommendations, the Secretary is required in section 264(b) to address at least the following: "(1) the rights that an individual who is the subject of individually identifiable information should have; (2) the procedures that should be established for the exercise of such rights; (3) the uses and disclosures of such information that should be authorized or required."

Since 1997, the NCVHS has focused almost exclusively on policies for the use and disclosure of individually identifiable health information with requirements to notify the health consumer, replacing rights of informed consent in many instances (U.S. DHHS, 1997). As part of this agenda, it intends to impose a unique health identifier for everyone so that private medical records can be easily accessed. A report titled "Records, Computers, and the Rights of Citizens" advised the Department of Health, Education and Welfare more than 25 years ago that, "in practice, the dangers inherent in establishing a standard universal identifier—without legal and social safeguards against the abuse of automated personal data systems— far outweigh any of its practical benefits" (U.S. Department of Health, Education, and Welfare, 1971). In response to the passage of HIPAA, Don Haines, the Legislative Counsel of the ACLU in Washington, D.C., has warned, "This bill will be remembered by Americans not as health care reform but as the thief who stole from us the privacy we deserve for our most confidential medical information" (Rosofsky, 1996, p. 2).

PERSON-DRIVEN PROTECTIONS OF HEALTH DATA

Americans do not want new rules permitting use and disclosure of identified health information. They want to be genuinely protected and their individual medical privacy *enhanced* through "the enforcement of long established privacy principles based on constitutional and statutory law, common law, the Hippocratic oath, the canons of medical ethics, and common sense" (*Health privacy issues,* 1997; Nagel, 1998, p. 1). In the computer age, the risks of data collection cannot be separated from the medical interventions that it documents. Therefore, policies and procedures for the protection of human subjects within a health data system, including the rights of privacy and confidentiality in research, evaluation, outcomes management, and quality assurance, should be mandated. In data integration activities, human subjects' protections accorded to research subjects should also apply. Following are some of the most important recommendations advanced by consumers and advocates to protect medical privacy. These privacy recommendations have emerged though consumer focus groups (Consumer/Survivor Mental Health Research and Policy Work Group, 1992; Trochim, Dumont, & Campbell, 1993), consumer-generated State Mental Health

Agency information policy documents (Kentucky Center for Mental Health Studies, Inc., 1998; Maine Department of Mental Health and Mental Retardation, 1993), and policy research (Campbell, 1998). Although these recommendations are particularly critical for protecting stigmatized populations, national polls indicate overwhelming support of all Americans for the protections discussed here (EPIC, 1999).

Informed Consent

At the core of privacy protection that health consumers want is the concept of informed consent. Consumers want to control the use of their records and want the sharing of health information to be voluntary. Therefore, any use of medical records in a person-driven system would require the consent of the consumer. The inclusion of consumer data within electronic databases of unified records or management information systems would also be voluntary and follow informed consent protocols. Some advocates have suggested that psychiatric records not be included in any system of electronic records (Rotenberg, 1994). Without specific informed consent, clinical records should not be retrospectively integrated into an information system. Data sharing and integration between agencies and systems may pose problems with regard to breaching both consumer and family confidentiality. An informed consent protocol regarding release of information between agencies or for storage in a data bank should be required before any data are synthesized or integrated.

Consent is contingent on the consumer's receiving information about the risks and benefits of the use and making an informed decision. Such protocols allow consumers to weigh not only the risks but also the benefits (e.g., better services, information to consumers, access to one's own records, payment for data) for providing information and to waive voluntarily certain protections or security measures for those benefits.

For consent to be truly informed, three factors must be considered: the quality of the information provided, the competence of the consumer to give consent, and the level of coercion to induce consent. Because informed consent protocols are usually written by researchers or administrators, conflicts of interest exist between the needs of the system and the needs of the individual consumer. To the researcher or administrator, the consent is sometimes viewed as an obstacle to convincing the consumer to agree to the data collection or use. Information in consent forms may be biased or inadequate. Furthermore, the request for consent to use medical records often comes from a busy clerk upon the consumer's admission to a service provider. Informed consent forms are buried in other paperwork, and people are routinely asked to "sign here" without explanation.

Surrogate consent may be appropriate depending on the competence and conservatorship status of the consumer. However, competence is not a precise legal term. In some states, the courts have ruled that involuntary patients in a psychiatric hospital are considered competent to refuse treatment.

Without consent, services can be denied under current laws. With consent, a person's records may be sent to a wide range of users who may not have adequate security. When health plans started demanding private information about patients, the Massachusetts Medical Society proposed perhaps the broadest privacy protections in the country. It said that patients should not be forced to give insurers blanket access to medical information in exchange for health coverage. "We don't believe in coerced consent. Right now, that's what patients give" (Stanley & Palosky, 1997b), announced the society's president. Any informed consent protocol that is designed to protect the consumer would have to remedy these problems to be effective.

The Option Out of the System

If services should not be denied to consumers who decline to give consent, then consumers need to be able to "opt out" of an electronic record system (i.e., the organization would keep a person's health records in paper form with some limited exceptions). Researchers have argued that incomplete data and bias could be introduced into outcome studies if this option were adopted. However, this claim is not based on any field research to determine how many consumers would opt out, or on whether the number would be constant, be based on respondent bias, or be reflective of organizational policies that would cause consumers to mistrust the information system. If the consumer believes that the benefits for inclusion outweigh the dangers and if the consumer trusts the organization to keep medical records secure, then few may take the option to stay out of the electronic information system. In fact, the number of consumers who opt out may be a good performance indicator of the information system.

Access

Consumers want full access to all personally identifiable medical records. No records should be kept secret from the consumer. Access to clinical and management information system data by service recipients should be supported with protocols developed for individuals to review and amend their records or to remove any inaccurate, irrelevant, or out-of-date information. Paternalistic medical systems consider access to personal health information part of the privilege and obligation of the doctor to protect the patient and often don't give patients access to their own records. Rather than build trust, this orientation weakens the bond between doctor and patient. Consumers fear what may be in their records, and misinformation has caused considerable harm in some cases.

Understandably, there is resistance in health organizations to allow service recipients to review their medical records. Information in the medical records could be misunderstood by the patient and in some cases, create greater liability risks for the health provider. Some mental health clinicians believe that a patient's progress could be harmed if he or she could read treatment notes. Such strategies as failure to notify a consumer of the right of review, excessive charges to the patient for copies, and lengthy waiting periods for records abound. The nature of electronic information systems has created opportunities to erect even greater barriers. Conversely, electronic information systems could just as easily be used to create opportunities for greater access and ease of access. With proper security, consumer access to personal medical records could help to improve the quality of the information in those records. Furthermore, consumer information used for policy and decision support, particularly de-identified, aggregated figures related to service information (costs, utilization, effectiveness, and consumer satisfaction with services), could be made public and accessible to all citizens. Therefore, electronic information systems could build in accountability to consumers at both the person level and the system level.

However, third-party access to medical records should be strictly limited to a need-to-know basis. Billing agencies should receive only encrypted information, and this information should be destroyed in a specified time period. Law enforcement officials should be required to obtain a warrant after showing a compelling government interest for each piece of information sought. Although privileged communications should never be disclosed, use of even the most general information to sell products to consumers without their written consent should also be banned. A drug store, for instance, would be prevented from contacting people who are taking psychiatric medications to pitch a new treatment or from selling their database to a pharmaceutical company.

Security

The methods used for data storage and distribution should be explicit, and storage and distribution practices should be audited periodically for compliance. Records in storage or transit should be encrypted. Audit trails should track each access to an individual's file. Policies and procedures should also be developed for the protection of consumer confidentiality when using cellular phones, facsimile machines, automated information systems with multiple access points, and other technologies that are used to store, analyze, and transmit information. Faxing has become an increasingly common means of sharing information, and although there are no hard numbers, it appears common for confidential medical records to be faxed to the wrong places. For example, one person, whose telephone number is one digit different from a diagnostic center's, received in a 2-year period faxes of medical records for 50–60 people, including 15-page medical histories. These faxes included patients' names, SSNs, and health insurance information. In some cases, there also were addresses and telephone numbers. When this person finally contacted the center and told them that they had the wrong number, she thought that she had solved the problem. Every hospital, lab, and doctor's office that regularly faxed to the center was contacted, but the faxes kept coming (Stanley & Palosky, 1997c). A consumer who is concerned about a health provider's faxing his or her medical records should be able to prohibit the provider from faxing. Also essential to security of records is proper training of personnel. All staff within an organization should be trained in the proper handling of confidential data and regularly evaluated on their performance.

Following the concept of "as much information as necessary, as little information as possible," another approach to protecting health information is to reduce the amount of information by collecting only what is essential. It is possible to reduce absolute risks to data security by collecting outcomes data on random samples rather than on entire recipient populations and by minimizing the amount of data actually collected per respondent. Furthermore, technologies such as virtual systems that use object technology may be able to replace data warehouses. These virtual systems would allow records to remain at their primary site and be linked only on request. Therefore, it is possible for the consumer, via an authorization protocol, to control the information that is available to the doctor (Work Group for Computerization of Behavioral Health and Human Services Records, 1997).

Privacy and security assurances under law should apply to all users of the information. When health information is transmitted to a third party, the recipient should be required to honor the same privacy and security assurances as the record's original holder. *The Final Report of the Legislative Survey of State Confidentiality Laws, with Specific Emphasis on HIV and Immunizations* suggested that the duty to protect data be "transferred simultaneously with the data, as would liability for violation of privacy or security standards" (Gostin, Lazzarini, & Flaherty, 1996).

Unique Identifier

Many systems call for the use of the SSN as a consumer identifier and assume that it is both possible and legitimate to convince consumers that the use would pose no risk or minimal risk to the privacy of an individual. However, consumer privacy under such systems cannot be totally safeguarded (*Protecting the privacy,* 1992; Ziglan, 1995). The widespread use of the SSN has seriously eroded personal privacy. The growing amounts of information that different organizations collect about a person can be linked because all of them use the same key to identify an individual. Chaum wrote, "This identifier-based approach perforce trades off security against individual liberties. The more information that organizations have, the less privacy and control people retain" (1992, p. 97). Personal security is also endangered through the use of the SSN as hackers and thieves routinely mine organizational databases looking for people to victimize. Given the stigma associated with mental illness and other disorders, using the SSN or any universal identifier not only poses substantial risks but also constitutes a barrier to access for those who are unwilling to take the risk. Using a person's SSN as a unique identifier should, therefore, be discouraged.

There are alternatives to using the SSN. One of the most promising is the "digital signature" on a smart credit-card-size computer containing memory and a microprocessor. The owner can control the data that are stored and exchanged by incorporating a keypad and display on the card. It would also be possible to incorporate fingerprint identification technology within the card itself to prevent anyone other than the owner from using it. The growing availability of such technologies argue against the use of a unique identification system and especially the use of the SSN. In a person-driven information system, concerns about identifiers would be acknowledged and validated. If unique identifiers are used, then only minimal information should be anchored to the identifier.

Data Removal

Once a person's health information is in a system file, it is usually there for life. This is true whether it is a paper file or an electronic file. However, electronic systems pose a greater danger because information is more easily accessible, regardless of age of the records and is accessible to a wide range of electronic network users. That means that if a person was in a psychiatric hospital, then a record of that admission would follow the consumer throughout his or her lifetime. It becomes a significant referential point for all clinical decisions in the future. In Maine, the court ordered the Department of Mental Health to notify all patients of the state psychiatric hospital during a certain time period of a legal decision regarding the department. Even though many people did not want to be found, records were pulled and merged with the motor vehicle license database. Letters went out bearing the Department of Mental Health return address on the envelope. As a result, some people were "outed" to their family and neighbors. For others, it was a difficult reminder of an episode that they wished to forget (J. Campbell, personal observation, August 1996). Mental health consumers want time limits on data storage to be specified and data destruction and removal protections to be developed and implemented when a person no longer receives mental health services. Procedures should also be developed and implemented for consumers to disenroll from an information system (except for minimal necessary data required to deliver services) without penalty. This is especially important when the information system has proved to have inadequate security or the organization has misused medical records.

Review Boards

Reviewing regulations imposed by review boards on health research reveals an implicit assumption that evaluation and outcomes data collection pose minimal risk to participants (Barrows & Clayton, 1996), but subjects report that there has been considerable abuse and that greater risks are involved than most researchers realize (Campbell & Frey, 1993; *Protecting the privacy,* 1992).

Policies and procedures similar to those for research subjects should be developed for the protection of human subjects within the data systems, and a review panel should evaluate prior to the use of consumer records the adequacy of such human subjects' protections in the collection, analysis, storage, and distribution of information. Data subjects' protections review panels should be based in the community. With Institutional Review Boards (IRBs), there is always the possibility for conflicts of interests as institutional culture and a shared ideology that is common to its membership tends to support the status quo. With local oversight shared by community members, especially by members of stigmatized or underrepresented populations, the interests of a review panel would be broadened and become responsive to the health privacy needs of individual consumers rather than health organizations and research institutions (Campbell, 1997c).

Laws and Penalties

Where laws guarantee to individuals medical privacy, exceptions proliferate and penalties are few. Donna E. Shalala, Secretary of the DHHS, announced, "Our private health information is being shared, collected, analyzed, and stored with fewer federal safeguards than our video store records. The way we protect the privacy of medical records right now is erratic at best, dangerous at worst" (Pear, 1997, p. A22)

There is much discussion about the constitutional right of privacy, but in practice, the Constitution has provided little support for medical record privacy claims in the United States. The Americans with Disabilities Act (ADA) of 1990 (PL 101-336) requires that medical information be kept confidential and separate from personnel files, but privacy harms are usually redressed through private actions, such as contract and tort, and sometimes by state agencies (Institute of Medicine, 1994). Every state and territory provides statutory protection for some types of personal health data maintained by a government agency. Forty-one states report statutory penalties for impermissible disclosures. Of these, 31 report criminal penalties, 18 report civil penalties, and 8 report both. Twenty-eight states provide statutory penalties for unauthorized disclosure of privately held health care information, twelve impose criminal penalties, nineteen create civil penalties, and three allow for both civil and criminal penalties (Gostin et al., 1996). Arrests and prosecutions are rare, however. For example, when a nurse showed to television reporters confidential mental health records from Charter Hospital Orlando South, state regulators suspended the nurse's license, and the hospital sued to stop the nurse and television reporters from calling patients who were named in the records. However, the nurse has not faced any criminal charges (Palosky & Stanley, 1997b). For penalties to be a deterrent against unauthorized disclosure, substantial criminal and civil fines should be imposed for actual or attempted unauthorized access, disclosure, or use of medical information. Individuals should be able to enforce rights and obtain damages and related costs in civil court. Furthermore, an independent agency should be created to conduct oversight and to enforce the provisions of any federal medical privacy law.

Retooling Human Technologies

In efforts to change medical privacy laws, policies, and practices, the marginalization of consumer concerns demands dialogue in collaboration with all of the data stakeholders. This is the first step in establishing an ethical center from which the challenges of the new information technologies may be engaged. In fact, public constituencies of people who have stigmatizing medical conditions should be sought out and supported as the jewels of a data-use reform process. Such an effort would go beyond developing law and policy to protect medical privacy, to resuscitating the body politic of a country deeply polarized by market forces, prejudice, and ethical ambiguity. It is clear that neither research protocols nor communication technologies that facilitate health data activities are simply mechanical, electronic, or intellectual tools and protocols that serve the needs of individuals and groups within society. Because reform in protecting medical privacy is limited by the attitudes and social relationships of those that research, manage, and deliver services, it follows that the source of new knowledge to guide the next generation of protections may lie in the incongruities between the perceptual and experiential framework of the "experts" and those who receive services.

By listening respectfully and treating data collection subjects with dignity, organizations have the power to bridge the differences between the system and service recipients and to generate new understandings (Campbell, 1996a). Instead of resisting criticism, they should welcome consumers and their families to the process, saying, "Gee, how can we improve?" Individually, each of us would also need to interrogate *a priori* assumptions about data collection and to bring to the table a reflexive understanding of the values, sensibilities, biases, and stereotypes that inform participation.

CONCLUSION

Those who handle health information must go beyond focusing on minimal compliance to privacy regulations to strive for excellence. This means rigorously applying the protections that already exist and monitoring their effectiveness to meet the concerns of health service recipients. To sustain data reform, environments in which whistle blowing is supported as part of a continuous quality improvement agenda need to be established. Medical privacy could also be fostered through development of a gold standard for management information system protocols. One starting point could be the Joint Commission on Accreditation of Healthcare Organizations, which now reviews management information systems and outcomes data collection in its standards, scoring, and decisions (Joint Commission on Accreditation of Healthcare Organizations, 1997). However, the accreditation process has limits because it monitors compliance to policies and procedures rather than the outcomes of such policies. Behavioral health delivery systems that support health data professionals who go beyond regulations to develop superior models should also be identified and that information disseminated. In particular, models that establish ongoing partnerships with health consumers or employ professionals with stigmatizing conditions should be sought out and supported. Finally, training people regarding medical privacy protections and ethics, especially when using case studies that exemplify the human dynamics of such issues, should also be built into human resource development activities (Campbell & Estroff, 1995).

At the heart of the mental health consumer movement is the belief that the goals of health care reform cannot be achieved without attending to the way individual decisions are made. In response to public demand for health organizations to be more open and accountable, a new vision for health care that is more humane, effective, and accountable can be achieved through the coordinated use of data by all stakeholders. Information technologies have the potential to humanize health care relationships by providing people with access to the most complete knowledge at the time of decision making, allowing recipients of medical services to partner effectively in care (Campbell, 1996a).

Business and government leaders must look at the context in which privacy protections operate, not just examine the regulations themselves (Campbell, 1997b). In the management of health data dehumanization naturally occurs. People forget that the objects of statistical inquiry are human beings. By gaining a humanistic focus, information technologies could be retooled to create an open architecture of health knowledge production and distribution. This development would present barriers to traditional data collection and use and, in some cases, would restrict the conduct of services research and data management. What is ironic is that these very actions could also lead to better information systems and encourage people to grow as ethical beings.

There is little hope that a data reform effort can really succeed if it is antagonistic to the cultural or social practices of those who exercise power within a system. There were human subjects' protections in place in Germany prior to World War II, and scientists justified the brutalization of people without much compunction, seeing them as less than human and expendable for scientific progress. However, anyone can prevent a rolled-up fax with the names of people committed to a psychiatric hospital from lying discarded on the floor of an administrative office. The seeds of a person-centered information system would grow from the heroics of everyday life, from people who begin to care enough about themselves as individual health consumers to stop making small compromises by looking the other way.

To prevent an escalation in the fight over access to and security of electronic patient health records and electronic management information systems, a fundamental change in corporate philosophy is needed. The focus on continual quality improvement of individual clinicians and the service system must be encouraged through the collaborative use of information by all stakeholders in the health delivery system. For consumers, fear can be driven out of electronic data collection by developing participatory action research initiatives, establishing data protections review boards with multistakeholder membership, and building trust and incentives for data sharing. As consumers become equal health information partners and data trustees with providers, they will recognize that even the best systems are not absolutely safe from security failures. Health information partnerships will enable the health care industry to move beyond issues of confidentiality and control of health records to embrace the principles of health informatics, or the education of the public by facilitating the distribution of health information. Only by making sure that people's privacy and confidentiality are protected and that people have access to needed health information—both clinical and administrative—can the mental health system effectively engage service recipients in building electronic health information networks.

To protect medical privacy, people must recognize that data reforms—including rules and regulations—are not out there waiting to be found or adjudicated, and society is not driven into the future by technological forces that stand outside social control. The future is contingent on each individual's looking with new eyes at policies regarding medical privacy and climbing for higher ground. In other words, it is the quality of ethical struggles to do the right thing, not particular outcomes, that will ultimately define health privacy protections in the computer age.

REFERENCES

American Civil Liberties Union. (1994). "Live and Let Live" Poll [On-line]. Available: http://www.epic.org/privacy/medical/polls.html

Americans with Disabilities Act (ADA) of 1990, PL 101-336, 42 U.S.C. 12101 *et seq.*

Applebaum, P., & Monahan, J. (1994, July 29). Brady bill's false step. *The Boston Globe,* 19.

Barrows, R., & Clayton, P. (1996). Privacy, confidentiality, and electronic medical records. *Journal of the American Informatics Association, 3*(2), 139–148.

Beisecker, A., & Beisecker, T. (1993). Using metaphors to characterize doctor–patient relationships: Paternalism versus consumerism. *Health Communication, 5*(1), 45–58.

Breitenstein, A., & Nagel, D. (1997, August 20). Keep your health history private. *The Los Angeles Times,* p. B7.

Burd, S. (1995, January 20). Adequate protection for human subjects? Researchers, advocates for mental patients clash over U.S. rules. *The Chronicle of Higher Education,* p. A29.

Campbell, J. (1996a). Toward collaborative mental health outcomes systems. *New Directions for Mental Health Services, 71,* 69–78.

Campbell, J. (1996b). Who owns the data? *Behavioral Healthcare Tomorrow, 5*(6), 49–51.

Campbell, J. (1997a). Ensuring ethical, accountable systems of care. In D. Evans & C. Harding (Eds.), *Decisions & dilemmas: Local-level managed mental health care* (pp. 21–26). Boulder, CO: Western Interstate Commission for Higher Education.

Campbell, J. (1997b). Privacy and confidentiality. In S. Moffic (Ed.), *The ethical way* (pp. 108–111). San Francisco: Jossey-Bass.

Campbell, J. (1997c). Reforming the IRB process: Towards new guidelines for quality and accountability in protecting human subjects. In A.E. Shamoo (Ed.), *Ethics in neurobiological research with human subjects: The Baltimore conference on ethics* (pp. 299–303). Amsterdam: Gordon and Breach Publishers.

Campbell, J. (1998). *The technical assistance needs of consumer/survivor stakeholder groups within state mental health agencies.* Alexandria, VA: National Technical Assistance Center for State Mental Health Planning.

Campbell, J., & Estroff, S. (1995). *Ethical issues in mental health services research: Technical report series.* Alexandria, VA: National Association of State Mental Health Program Directors Research Institute.

Campbell, J., & Frey, E. (1993). *Humanizing decision support systems: Report to the Mental Health Statistics Improvement Program (MHSIP).* Rockville, MD: Center for Mental Health Services.

Chaum, D. (1992). Achieving electronic privacy. *Scientific American, 267*(2) 96–101.

Consumer/Survivor Mental Health Research and Policy Work Group. (1992). *Reports 1, 2, 3.* Fort Lauderdale, FL: Center for Mental Health Services Knowledge Exchange Network.

Electronic Privacy Information Center. (1999). *Medical privacy public opinion polls* [On-line]. Available: http://www.epic.org/privacy/medical/polls.html

Equifax "Harris Consumer Privacy Survey" [On-line]. Available: http://www.epic.org/privacy/medical/polls.html

Flores, G. (June 2, 1997). Testimony. National Committee on Vital and Health Statistics. San Francisco, CA.

Gates, J. (1998, Summer). Privacy and confidentiality of health information. *Treatment Today, 10*(2), 7.

Gostin, L., Lazzarini, Z., & Flaherty, K. (1996). *Legislative survey of state confidentiality laws, with specific emphasis on HIV and immunization.*

(Final report presented to the U.S. Centers for Disease Control and Prevention, The Council of State and Territorial Epidemiologists, and the Task Force for Child Survival and Development, Carter Presidential Center [On-line]). Available: http://www.epic.org/privacy/medical/cdc survey.html

Gostin, L., Lazzarini, Z., Neslund, V., & Osterholm, M. (1996). The public health information infrastructure: A national review of law on health information privacy. *Journal of the American Medical Association, 275*(24), 1921–1927.

Hayden, T. (1988). *Reunion: A memoir.* New York: Random House.

Health Insurance Portability and Accountability Act of 1996, PL 104-191, 42 U.S.C. 201 §§ *et seq.*

Health privacy issues: Hearings before the Subcommittee on Privacy and Confidentiality of the National Committee on Vital and Health Statistics. (1997, February 19). (testimony of Denise Nagel).

Institute of Medicine. (1994). *Health data in the information age: Use, disclosure, and privacy.* Washington, DC: National Academy Press.

Katz, J. (1972). *Experimentation with human beings.* New York: Russel Sage Foundation.

Kentucky Center for Mental Health Studies, Inc. (1998). *From the KCMHS Notebook: Consumer Guidelines for Research and Data Management.* Lexington: Author.

Maine Department of Mental Health and Mental Retardation. (1993). *Draft policy on privacy and confidentiality of mental health data.* Augusta: Office of Research, Quality Assurance and Information Services.

Nagel, D. (1998). Outcomes, paving the way to loss of health privacy? *P/C 2000, 3*(2), 1, 3.

National Committee on Vital and Health Statistics. (1997, June 24–25). *Minutes.* Washington, DC: U.S. Department of Health and Human Services.

Ovellette, P. (1993). *The deus machine.* New York: Pocket Star Books.

Palosky, C., & Stanley, D. (1997a, February 15). Famous breaches of medical privacy. *The Tampa Tribune* [On-line]. Available: http://www.tampa trib.com/reports/medical/home.htm

Palosky, C., & Stanley, D. (1997b, February 19). Computer full of secrets. *The Tampa Tribune* [On-line]. Available: http://www.tampatrib.com/ reports/medical/home.htm

Palosky, C., & Stanley, D. (1997c, March 2). Readers fear medical secrets a tool for firing. *The Tampa Tribune* [On-line]. Available: http://www. tampatrib.com/reports/medical/home.htm

Pear, R. (1997, August 10). Clinton to back a law on patient privacy. *The New York Times,* p. A22.

Petersen, C. (1995). PCA takes on Florida's government over disclosure. *Managed Healthcare, 5*(8), 10–13.

Petrila, J. (1996, March). Ethics: The core values of privacy and confidentiality. *P/C 2000, 1*(1), 1–3.

Protecting the privacy of social security numbers and records. Hearings before the Subcommittee on Social Security and Family Policy, Committee on Finance, Senate, 102d Cong., pro forma Sess. (1992). (testimony of Marc Rotenberg).

Robitscher, J. (1981). *The powers of psychiatry.* Boston: Houghton Mifflin.

Rosofsky, I. (1996). The law: Assaults on privacy in Kennedy-Kassebaum. *Practice Management Monthly, 4*(10), 1–2.

Rotenberg, M. (October, 1994). *Keynote address: Seizing the Opportunity: The power of health information.* The American Health Information Management Association national convention, Las Vegas, NV.

Stanley, D., & Palosky, C. (1997a, February 15). Health information industry embraces technology. *The Tampa Tribune* [On-line]. Available: http://www.tampatrib.com/reports/medical/home.htm

Stanley, D., & Palosky, C. (1997b, February 19). Patients should control data, advocates say. *The Tampa Tribune* [On-line]. Available: http://www.tampatrib.com/reports/medical/home.htm

Stanley, D., & Palosky, C. (1997c, February 28). Fax drops records in her lap. *The Tampa Tribune* [On-line]. Available: http://www.tampatrib.com/reports/medical/home.htm

Stanley, D., & Palosky, C. (1997d, March 2). Employees at risk. *The Tampa Tribune* [On-line]. Available: http://www.tampatrib.com/reports/medical/home.htm

The Joint Commission on Accreditation of Healthcare Organizations. (1997). *Comprehensive accreditation manual for behavioral health care.* Oakbrook Terrace, IL: Author.

Trochim, W., Dumont, J., & Campbell, J. (1993). *A report for the state mental health agency profiling system: Mapping mental health outcomes from the perspective of consumers/survivors. Technical report series.* Alexandria, VA: National Association of State Mental Health Program Directors.

U.S. Department of Health and Human Services (U.S. DHHS). (1997, September). *Confidentiality of individually-identifiable health information, recommendations of the Secretary of Health and Human Services, pursuant to section 264 of the Health Insurance Portability and Accountability Act of 1996.* Washington, DC: Author.

Wedding, D., Topolski, J., & McGaha, A. (1995). Maintaining the confidentiality of computerized mental health outcome data. *The Journal of Mental Health Administration, 22*(3), 237–244.

Weisburd, D. (Ed.). (1994). Ethics in neurobiological research with human subjects. *The Journal of the California Alliance for the Mentally Ill, 5*(1).

Work Group for Computerization of Behavioral Health and Human Services Records. (1997, May). *Towards the consumer-focused behavioral health and human services record.* Unpublished report.

World Book Year Book. (1974). Chicago: Field Enterprises Educational Corporation.

Ziglan, A. (1995). *Confidentiality and appropriate uses of data.* Rockville, MD: Center for Mental Health Services.

Zinn, H. (1990). *A people's history of the United States.* New York: Harper Perennial.

3

Families' Perspectives on Confidentiality in the Treatment of Mental Illness

Harriet P. Lefley

Breaches of confidentiality in the treatment of mental illness may involve disclosure of status (i.e., that someone has a psychiatric condition) and disclosure of information. Families have concerns in both domains. Families fear that any disclosure of psychiatric history or diagnosis may affect the availability of insurance, jobs, housing, and educational opportunities; generate vulnerability to criminal charges; and generally diminish a person's quality of life. They fear that the requirements of managed care and multiple access points to information greatly facilitate such disclosure.

Not all disclosure is detrimental, however. A focus of this chapter is on the confidentiality of records of adults with mental illness as they relate to the family relationship and on modes of distinguishing those aspects of information that may be beneficial rather than harmful to the consumer.

UNIQUE ASPECTS OF THE FAMILY RELATIONSHIP

The family relationship is uniquely different from that of clinicians, third-party payers, or citizens concerned with the confidentiality of psychiatric records. From the beginning, background information is solicited from family members, and their input contributes to developing case histories and medical records. The flow of information typically is unilateral; there is little reciprocal exchange from clinicians because of confidentiality guidelines. In many cases, however, the family plays an important lifetime role in caregiving. Pragmatic needs for information must be considered when families are the primary caregivers or the major support system for a person with a psychiatric disability.

Several aspects of disclosure of status are also unique to the family relationship. First, in contrast to mental health staff or other concerned individuals, there is personal emotional investment of family members when breaches of confidentiality evoke distress in a loved one. When a person's psychiatric condition is disclosed, families share the anguish and adverse consequences that may result from stigmatization and deprivation of needed opportunities for employment or higher education. Family members' lives may be directly affected when breaches of confidentiality lead to an individual's demoralization, giving up, and increased dependence on caregivers. Families also have the unique problem of entwined identity, discussed next.

Entwined Identity

Having an entwined identity means that family members cannot disclose their status as relatives of a person with a psychiatric disorder without revealing information that is not theirs alone. Many family members prefer openness, but a far more important consideration is whether they breach confidentiality by sharing their own status. Many family members belong to organizations or support groups identified with mental illness, and some are sought by the media to tell their stories. Families often have difficulties obtaining timely help for a person who is experiencing a psychotic episode or engaging in self-destructive behaviors. They must cope with a treatment system that is sometimes unresponsive and inaccessible. Many would be willing to talk about their personal experiences to help correct deficiencies of the system. Unless the person's condition is publicly known, however, family members fear that they may jeopardize the reputation or aspirations of a loved one. They feel that they must seek consent before telling their own stories. Entwined identity thus may prevent some families from educating the public by sharing their own experiences with system deficits or social barriers or by highlighting elements of recovery because such a discussion may compromise their relative's right to privacy.

These considerations suggest that confidentiality is a concept that is both elastic and context bound. Types of information disclosure may range from second-order identification of status to a patient's specific diagnosis and prognosis. From the family's perspective, confidentiality may lead to negative or positive consequences.

In certain contexts, the sharing of information may be helpful, whereas the withholding of information may be harmful. Determining the parameters of confidentiality is particularly important when family members are the major caregivers and are involved on a day-to-day basis with a relative's progress.

Deinstitutionalization and Family Roles in Caregiving

Deinstitutionalization, the emptying of mental hospitals, brought families into a caregiving role for which they were untrained and unprepared and from which they had been functionally excluded. Formerly, patients spent many years living away in large, isolated institutions. Today, they live in the community. From a variety of studies, it is estimated that, on average, 50% of people with severe mental illness live at home with family caregivers (Lefley, 1996). Percentages tend to vary by ethnicity; ethnic minority groups are more likely to keep the person at home. In one study, for example, 84% of Hispanic and 59% of African American clients were living with family members, versus 44% of European Americans (Guarnaccia, 1998). Even when clients live in housing affiliated with mental health programs, research shows that family members provide ongoing social, emotional, and financial support (Clark & Drake, 1994).

Despite these responsibilities, families continue to be hampered by outmoded psychiatric theories and practices that have long denied them communication with and information from mental health professionals. Strict confidentiality rules are embedded in the regulations of professional associations and the institutions in which professionals practice. Families are treated very differently in the medical sector, where family education is standard. In the psychiatric sector, despite a dozen rigorous studies showing the benefits to the patient of family education (Dixon & Lehman, 1995), families continue to receive little information and almost no formal training in illness management (Dixon et al., 1999).

PSYCHIATRIC THEORIES AND CONFIDENTIALITY

The theories behind certain psychiatric practices have hindered family members' abilities as caregivers and have distorted principles of confidentiality in the doctor–patient relationship.

Communication with Families

For many years, psychiatric theories of the etiology of major mental illnesses, such as schizophrenia or bipolar disorder, were predicated on models of defective parenting or traumatic events in childhood. Prior to the advent of psychotropic medications, the major treatment approach was psychodynamic psychotherapy. Transference, the projection of relationships with past authority figures onto the therapist, is an essential aspect of achieving a corrective emotional experience in psychotherapy. The therapeutic alliance of therapist and patient becomes a means of healing emotional damage. In this treatment model, communication with families is precluded because it may contaminate transference, disrupt the therapeutic alliance, and impede healing. Giving information to families is viewed as a gross breach of confidentiality that will be perceived by the patient as a betrayal of trust.

This model is still applicable to many emotional problems, but it is inappropriate and potentially damaging in the case of major psychiatric disorders such as schizophrenia, major affective disorders, and other diagnoses with demonstrated neurobiological substrates. These conditions typically are treated with psychotropic medications, behavioral rehabilitative techniques, and supportive counseling rather than with psychodynamic approaches. The etiological theories have largely been discredited, but the rationale for communication barriers has been maintained. Regardless of diagnosis, severity of illness, dependency status, or therapeutic modality, this essentially psychodynamic paradigm has extended to most mental health practice.

Clinicians in training are still taught by some mentors not to communicate with families, and they are not taught any ethical responsibility to relieve families' bewilderment and pain. Professional education programs generally have been unconcerned with the confusion, anguish, and fears of patients' distressed relatives and have been ignorant of the effects of rejecting families' overtures for information. It is unfortunate that clinicians' mandates to do no harm bypass their patients' relatives because this can have severe clinical consequences for the patient as well.

A patient is admitted to the hospital after his first psychotic episode. He is assigned to a psychiatric resident who refuses to return the family's pleading calls for information. The social worker is on vacation, and the nurse will inform them only that the patient is doing as well as can be expected. The patient is discharged to the family with no diagnosis and no further information except for a prescription and a follow-up appointment 1 month later. The patient is eager to get back to his interrupted college courses. He immerses himself in studying and signs up for additional credits to make up for lost time with enthusiastic reinforcement from the family. When he experiences decompensation and has to be readmitted, the family complains that the hospital failed to educate them about pressure and the possibility of relapse. The psychiatric resident admits that she would have been happy to do this, but, "My supervisor told me never to return the family's calls."

Fortunately, practice guidelines are changing. Psychiatric guidelines for inpatient care now call for contact with families and family education. State plans suggest families' involvement in long-term treatment planning. There is still confusion about caregivers' roles in outpatient treatment, and there are few mandates or guidelines for families' involvement in private-sector care.

A psychiatrist refuses to answer calls from a patient's family, even though they pay his fees. He is rather peeved at these calls because he considers himself progressive and had long ago informed them of the ground rules regarding communication and confidentiality. The mother is concerned because the patient, who is taking monoamine oxidase inhibitors, has a severe cold and has been taking excessive doses of over-the-counter decongestants. The patient's blood pressure has shown an alarming rise, and the mother wants to know whether there is an interaction with the neuroleptics. Finally, she is forced to call a primary care physician, who informs her that indeed there may be a connection. In disclosing the psychotropic medication, however, she has been forced to breach the confidentiality of her daughter's diagnosis.

Distinguishing Content Areas

Obviously, there are differences between private disclosures and information that is essential for illness management. Families have long claimed that they do not want to know the intimate details of relatives' thoughts and feelings (e.g., McElroy, 1990) but that they do need to know the diagnosis so that they can research it and become knowledgeable enough for long-term treatment planning. Families need to know about medications and their anticipated behavioral effects, potential interactive and side effects, and how to ensure medication compliance without angering their relatives or encroaching on their autonomy. Families want to be able to assess accountability and what they can appropriately expect in the way of social interactions, manners, household responsibilities, work, and participation in rehabilitation programs. They want information on how to determine prodromal cues of decompensation, defuse psychotic flare-ups, and avert crises. This may require more time than professionals are willing or able to invest. It may—and should—require formal family education offered by hospitals, clinics, community mental health centers, and similar agencies. However, many of these issues may be worked out in collaborative sessions in which clinicians, families, and clients work out the parameters and boundaries of confidential information.

Petrila and Sadoff (1992) suggested that the mental health professions should seriously reexamine the application of rigid confidentiality rules, particularly when they compromise the ability of families to function effectively as caregivers. They also pointed out that there may be legal liability when mental health providers fail to share critical information with families, and this leads to adverse consequences such as murder or physical violence. They cited a case in which a hospital was negligent because it failed to inform the family that their relatives' noncompliance with neuroleptic medications may lead to regression and violence. In another case of severe injury to a family member, the court stated that the clinician should have warned the family of the patient's potential for danger and provided instructions about what to do if the patient's condition deteriorated. Petrila and Sadoff (1992) stated that although some clinicians might consider this a breach of confidentiality, from a risk management perspective it clearly is better to enlist the family as an ally rather than keep them in the dark. From both clinical and ethical perspectives as well, it makes little sense to maintain confidentiality when doing so results in danger to another and to consequences that will ruin a patient's life.

PRIVACY AND CONFIDENTIALITY: WHO OWNS THE INFORMATION?

In the mental health context, the right to privacy typically connotes protection from disclosure of information that is solely the concern of the individual involved. In the main, revealing the information meets no pressing social need and does not affect the personal interests of others.

The right to confidentiality, however, derives from a situation in which privacy has already been breached because it involves information to which at least two parties are privy. The second party is enjoined from disclosing to others information regarding the first party, whether by law, ethics, or professional convention. These constraints are operative regardless of whether the information affects the personal interests of the potential recipient. Clinicians may share information only in unusually threatening circumstances and only to protect third parties from harm (*Tarasoff v. Regents of the University of California*, 1976).

The individual generally determines whether to open doors to her or his privacy. The boundaries of confidentiality, however, can be defined by others. This is particularly true in the mental health field. Clinicians and agencies can make unilateral decisions not to share information that they define as confidential without involving the individual in the decision. They may also withhold information from the individuals themselves.

The question of who owns the information is the subject of a lawsuit filed by a Florida attorney who sought access to her medical records for a brief psychiatric hospitalization and found the diagnosis blotted out (Rafinski, 1997). Although medical records generally are accessible in Florida, they can be withheld from individuals who have been treated for mental or emotional problems. This lawsuit seeks to overturn the exemption that allows psychiatrists to deny records to their patients. The rationale for denying patients access to their records is that psychiatric patients have distorted thinking and may misinterpret what is written, with harmful results. Until the issue is resolved, Florida psychiatrists may elect to share or deny records, and patients may continue to find it difficult to obtain psychiatric hospital records after they are discharged.

The implicit rationale for withholding records is to protect the patient from harm. Individuals with psychiatric diagnoses vary enormously in level of functioning, in the severity and chronicity of their disorders, and particularly in their cognitive capacity and judgment. It is beyond the scope of this chapter to address the therapeutic parameters and implications of a paternalistic stance that may be necessary for some patients and offensive to others. A representative of the American Psychiatric Association Committee for Privacy and Law has stated that most patients do get their records and that only a tiny minority are denied for good reasons (Rafinski, 1997). The main point here is that clinicians or hospitals essentially own not only the decision to disclose but also the information itself, and they can withhold it from the people whose lives and destinies are most vitally invested in that information.

Many families have experienced the power of clinicians and institutions to make critical decisions regarding the sharing of any kind of information with patients. The files of the Office of Homeless and Missing Persons of the National Alliance for the Mentally Ill are full of stories of families who tried to track down missing relatives only to be told by a hospital or an institution that they could not disclose whether the person was even there. Clearly, this is a protective practice meant to prevent the identification of psychiatric patients to unknown callers. However, there appears to be no mandate to share the relatives' calls or even to take down relevant information in case the person is there and wants reunification. The decision for relaying a family's inquiry may be made by the staff member who answers the call or perhaps by the clinician to whom it may be conveyed. If they decide against disclosure, however, then the person to whom this decision is central may be excluded from the loop.

In several cases, anxious families have later learned that their loved ones were indeed in a certain place but were not informed of their relatives' call (see Lefley, Neuhring, & Bestman, 1992). Clinicians may make this judgment if they believe that the inquiry may be disturbing or that it is in the patient's best interest not to reunite her or him with the family on whom she or he is dependent, but withholding information from a patient is a gross misuse of confidentiality, both ethically and therapeutically. It disempowers the person who should be the decision maker, and it reinforces dependence by substituting the judgment of another.

Zipple, Langle, Spaniol, and Fisher (1990) suggested some remedial procedures for release of information. They noted that when a person is discharged from a hospital or transferred to another program, the sharing of relevant information is expected by the receiving agency. They recommended similar client release forms to share information with family caregivers. "In our experience, when the client is approached in a supportive way by a practitioner who believes in the value of involving families, most disabled consumers are willing to grant some degree of access to family members" (Zipple et al., 1990, p. 541).

This is extremely important for therapeutic as well as practical reasons. People with mental illness are disempowered by the limitations of their condition but even more by their intrinsic status of dependence on society, the treatment system, and their caregivers. Many are angry at their lot, rail at their fate, and project their feelings of rage and helplessness onto those with whom they are most intimately involved. Some clinicians have taken these expressions at face value and reinforced separation from families. Others have realized the underlying reasons and, by putting ownership of information and decision making in the patients' hands, created a more equitable relationship and facilitated rebonding with family members.

As clinicians increasingly are mandated to involve families in treatment and discharge planning, the need to ask patients to share relevant information puts ownership of confidentiality back into the hands of the patient, or consumer. There are many ways of conferring with consumers about the boundaries of information and of honoring their wishes in ways that will be acceptable to them and to the family. If patients do not want the involvement of an obviously concerned family, then the issues should be explored. Very often, as Zipple et al. (1990) suggested, consumers may be persuaded to change their minds. It may be highly therapeutic to bring all family members together for mutual decision making. The consumer and the family members can discuss practical issues of aftercare, long-term housing, financial support, and medication management and agree on strategies for solving other problems that may arise.

Confidentiality has often erected barriers between patients and families. Family involvement becomes a way of reintegrating consumers with their major support systems. Most important, it accords consumers the fundamental respect of owning their own information and controlling its uses.

Confidentiality and Family Therapy

There are many cases, particularly with young adults, in which families have been informed that their relatives could not be treated unless they themselves entered family therapy. McElroy (1990), a professor of psychiatric nursing, has written about ethical and confidentiality issues involved in what she perceives as essentially coerced treatment. She also deplores families' being used in clinical training without informed consent. In one case, the parents of a hospitalized patient were required to participate in family therapy, although they strongly indicated their reluctance. After making intimate disclosures for at least 10 minutes, they were informed that they were being observed by students through a one-way mirror and that their words were being recorded. In another case, after being asked to travel 30 miles to confer with a consultant, parents were informed that the session was being videotaped and that 11 professionals would be observing. They were not given this information until they had arrived at the session, and they were afraid of the consequences if they objected (McElroy, 1990).

In both cases, the families had legitimate complaints of coercion, lack of informed consent, and invasion of privacy. Even if families have the right to refuse their own participation in treatment, coercion is implicit simply in the knowledge that their loved one's treatment may be affected by their refusal. There is also the question of the uses of the information gained by strangers' observations through a one-way mirror. A study in a large hospital indicated that as many as 75 people may have a legitimate need to have access to a patient's medical information (Fleck, 1986), but this access is in the interest of helping the patient. The breaches of confidentiality in the previously cited cases were not to help the patient but to train future family therapists. Moreover, the students were being trained in what the writer, a clinical educator, believed to be an *in*appropriate and *counter* therapeutic model for those particular cases.

This is the other side of the entwined identity issue. Obviously, there are disclosures other than those of the patient that must be protected. The confidentiality issues raised when patients and families are under observation by clinical trainees and the extra vulnerabilities of being observed by multiple viewers are areas that have yet to be fully explored. McElroy (1990) suggested detailed guidelines for procedures and objectives that will protect patients and ensure that families are sufficiently informed before they give consent for sharing personal information with strangers.

CULTURAL ASPECTS OF FAMILIES AND CONFIDENTIALITY

The entwined interests of patients and families are further suggested in the cross-cultural literature in mental illness. International studies indicate that members of traditional, group-oriented cultures throughout the world, as well as many ethnic groups in the United States, do not view individuals' rights to privacy as separate from those of the groups to which they belong (Triandis, 1995). In contrast to mainstream American culture, with its emphasis on the primacy of individual rights, traditional ethnic groups tend to be bewildered by the separation of the rights of individuals from the welfare of their kinship network (see Lefley, 1998, and Triandis, 1995, for research overview). In the medical sector, many physicians have discovered that families from traditional cultures believe that a diagnosis of cancer or a poor prognosis should be conveyed to the family rather than to the patient. The family will then assume the caregiving tasks necessary for healing, survival, or a dignified death.

Most anthropologists agree that in such cultures it would be highly inappropriate not to involve the family in all matters concerning a patient's health and welfare, particularly in the treatment of psychopathology (see Good, 1992). Two noted psychiatrists affiliated with the World Health Organization pointed out the following:

> Notions regarding confidentiality differ across cultures. In some settings patients assume that any information conveyed to the clinician is a private and individual matter. Indeed, the laws and state apparatus may reinforce this belief. . . . In other societies the standard may be quite different. It may be assumed that anything conveyed to the clinician might be shared with the family, clan leader, or elder. In such set-

tings, the unit of confidentiality may be the family rather than the individual. (Westermeyer & Janca, 1997, p. 302)

Many immigrant and ethnic minority groups in the United States share these values, and, as previously demonstrated, research shows that in these groups people with mental illness are most likely to be living with family caregivers (Guarnaccia, 1998). Yet in many cases, information that is readily available to managed care and other third-party payers is still denied to those who are most intimately involved with a patient's daily welfare.

RETHINKING CONFIDENTIALITY

With advances in technology, it has become increasingly difficult for individuals to maintain ownership of their own life histories. There are multiple access points to privileged information and ever fewer protections against breaches of privacy and confidentiality. Such breaches potentially have adverse effects on the lives of people with mental illness. Because confidential records are increasingly sieve-like and cannot be safeguarded, they require legal protections against the negative results of disclosure even more than against the disclosure itself. There must be accessible legal aid to enforce the provisions of the Americans with Disabilities Act (ADA) of 1990 (PL 101-336) when breaches of confidentiality lead to discrimination because of a history of mental illness.

Privacy and confidentiality are cultural constructs whose maintenance generally has been considered helpful for individuals with mental illness. The down side is that cultural and clinical conventions based on secrecy reinforce stigma by implying that mental illness is too shameful to talk about. Secrecy heightens the anxieties that surround disclosure. Individuals and society pay a price for maintaining a veil of secrecy that is becoming increasingly permeable in mental health care (Sabin, 1997).

The increasing permeability of confidential records may constitute an opportunity for reframing mental illness in the public's mind. There are practical and psychological benefits to disclosure. First, greater openness can generate more awareness of different categories and types of mental illness, particularly as new efforts to confine criminals such as sexual offenders in mental hospitals are initiated. It is important for the public to have access to information that distinguishes noncriminal people with brain disorders from people who are a menace to the public good. The public should also become educated about treatment and recovery potential and about the enriching contributions of many people with depression and bipolar disorder to our political, scientific, and cultural histories (Jamison, 1993). All of these diagnoses should become identified with pride and mastery of adversity rather than with stigma.

Hiding a psychiatric history means accepting and perpetuating the fearful attributions of the outside world. Psychiatric conditions are very heterogeneous, and a curtain of confidentiality can blur diagnostic distinctions, mask capabilities, and imply a lower level of functioning than is actually the case. Many consumers and family members have found greater personal strength and an attentive audience when they have talked openly about their experiences. The pages of some scientific journals, such as *Schizophrenia Bulletin* and *Psychiatric Services,* now have regular sections for experiential accounts of mental illness. Personal accounts are highly edifying to professionals and lead to greater public understanding and respect. A climate of openness can bring patients to a greater appreciation of their own coping capabilities and can reduce the societal and self-stigmatizations that have made confidentiality necessary.

CONCLUSION

In this chapter, which has focused on the case records of adults with severe and persistent mental illness, categories and ownership of information have been discussed as well as appropriate recipients and uses of information. Families' perspectives on confidentiality have been assessed in cultural and historical contexts. Confidentiality conventions that are based on outmoded psychiatric theories have become maladaptive with increased family caregiving needs for information. It has been emphasized that families want information for illness management, not for invading their relatives' privacy.

In cases of potential violence, there may be legal requirements for clinicians to notify families. In most cases, however, clients themselves can be encouraged to share those areas of information that are relevant to their families' provision of knowledgeable caregiving or support.

The process of working out the boundaries of confidentiality can bond families and clients in mutual decision making and give clients some needed power over their lives. Such sharing ultimately may lead to better illness control and stabilization and a renewed capacity of consumers to make their own decisions. Finally, reconceptualizing confidentiality may lead to destigmatizing a condition that should be associated with triumph over adversity rather than with shame and secrecy.

REFERENCES

Americans with Disabilities Act (ADA) of 1990, PL 101-336, 42 U.S.C. §§ 12101 *et seq.*

Clark, R.E., & Drake, R.E. (1994). Expenditure of time and money of families of people with severe mental illness and substance abuse disorders. *Community Mental Health Journal, 30,* 145–163.

Dixon, L., & Lehman, A. (1995). Family interventions in schizophrenia. *Schizophrenia Bulletin, 21,* 631–643.

Dixon, L., Lyles, A., Scott, J., Lehman, A., Postrada, L., Goldman, H., et al. (1999). Services to families of adults with schizophrenia: From treatment recommendations to dissemination. *Psychiatric Services, 50,* 233–238.

Fleck, L. (1986). Confidentiality: Moral obligation or outmoded concept? *Health Progress, 61,* 17–20.

Good, B.J. (1992). Culture and psychopathology: Directions for psychiatric anthropology. In T. Schwartz, G.M. White, & C.A. Lutz (Eds.), *New directions in psychological anthropology* (pp. 181–205). London: Cambridge University Press.

Guarnaccia, P.J. (1998). Multicultural experiences in family caregiving: A study of African American, European American, and Hispanic American families. *New Directions for Mental Health Services, 77,* 45–61.

Jamison, K.R. (1993). *Touched with fire: Manic-depressive illness and the artistic temperament.* Detroit: The Free Press.

Lefley, H.P. (1996). *Family caregiving in mental illness.* Thousand Oaks, CA: Sage Publications.

Lefley, H.P. (1998). Families, culture, and mental illness: Constructing new realities. *Psychiatry, 61,* 335–355.

Lefley, H.P., Neuhring, E., & Bestman, E.W. (1992). Homelessness and mental illness: A transcultural family perspective. In H.R. Lamb, L. Bachrach, & F.I. Kass (Eds.), *Treating the homeless mentally ill.* Washington, DC: American Psychiatric Press.

McElroy, E. (1990). Ethical and legal considerations for interviewing families of the seriously mentally ill. In H.P. Lefley & D.L. Johnson (Eds.), *Families as allies in treatment of the mentally ill: New directions for mental health professionals* (pp. 173–193). Washington, DC: American Psychiatric Press.

Petrila, J.P., & Sadoff, R.L. (1992). Confidentiality and the family as caregiver. *Hospital & Community Psychiatry, 43,* 136–139.

Rafinski, K. (1997, July 5). Protecting patients or discrimination? Woman sues for access to her psychiatric records. *The Miami Herald,* pp. A1, A25.

Sabin, J.E. (1997). What confidentiality standards should we advocate for in mental health care, and how should we do it? *Psychiatric Services, 40,* 35–41.

Tarasoff v. Regents of the University of California, 17 Cal 3rd 425; 551 P.2d 334 (1976).

Triandis, H. (1995). *Individualism and collectivism.* San Francisco: Westview.

Westermeyer, J., & Janca, A. (1997). Language, culture, and psychopathology: Conceptual and methodological issues. *Transcultural Psychiatry, 34,* 291–311.

Zipple, A.M., Langle, S., Spaniol, L., & Fisher, H. (1990). Client confidentiality and the family's need to know: Strategies for resolving the conflict. *Community Mental Health Journal, 26,* 533–545.

4

Privacy Issues in Child Mental Health Services

Gary B. Melton

Readers of this book are sure to come to one common conclusion: Privacy issues in mental health (and, for that matter, other contexts) are complex. At one level (perhaps the most obvious one), the complexity is a direct reflection of 1) the number of parties involved in privacy issues and 2) the conflicts among their interests. When privacy issues arise in regard to children and adolescents,[1] the complexity and confusion are multiplied. The cast of parties and interests is legion and well known:

- Insurers and health care administrators want to obtain information that may be used in monitoring the quantity and quality of services and determining the "risk" (in effect, the costs) associated with a particular current or prospective client.
- Providers want to protect the confidentiality of clinical information so that the trust necessary for a therapeutic relationship will not be disrupted, and they do not want their time for healing patients (and making money) disrupted by demands to report all that they have done and learned in the course of service delivery.
- Clients want to retain control over personal information and to avoid the embarrassment, stigma, and discrimination that may result from its disclosure, but they also want to ensure that their

---

[1] For convenience, except when developmental distinctions are directly relevant, "children" and "childhood" will be used in the remainder of this chapter to include "adolescents" and "adolescence."

services are effective, safe, and, therefore, monitored. They also want their providers' paperwork minimized so that therapists have maximum time for service delivery and so that costs do not rise.

- The public wants to ensure that the delivery of health services is efficient, that the quality of care is acceptable, that people with mental health problems are not deterred from seeking treatment by threats to their privacy, and that information needed to protect the public health and safety is available to relevant authorities (including researchers) and potential victims.

As this brief litany indicates, the conflicts of interest among parties are vast, and the parties themselves typically have mixed and often conflicting interests. Moreover, the strength of the numerous interests may vary across time and situations because of the state of knowledge. For example, the conventional wisdom about the desirability of absolute confidentiality of information about people's HIV status has changed as the probability that the information could be used for a beneficent purpose (e.g., treatment to extend life and reduce suffering) has increased.

The complexity is not simply a matter, however, of the number of parties, the diversity of their interests, and the uncertainty of clinical prediction and treatment. The *concept* of privacy is notoriously obtuse. The following events that we all would agree have something to do with privacy are remarkable for their lack of obvious common elements: being watched while one is undressing; having one's mail read; being asked one's income; being told to describe one's dreams; having one's house entered without permission; having one's purchase record sold by one company to another; and being required by an employer or a school official to be fingerprinted, provide a urine sample, or take a personality test.

The diversity is even more remarkable when one considers the nature of the incidents (tabloid reports about the wives of Justice-to-be Louis Brandeis and his law partner) that led to the ultimate explication of the construct of privacy in a dazzling array of constitutional, common-law, and statutory contexts. Brandeis's succinct, colloquial description of privacy as "the right to be let alone" (*Olmstead v. United States,* 1928, dissenting opinion of Justice Brandeis; Warren & Brandeis, 1890) captured the common element in intrusions on privacy: a gut sense of personal violation. One might say that the concept of privacy is so subjective that "I know it when I see it" or, more precise, that "I know it when I *feel* it."

In considering questions about the limits of privacy, it is worth keeping in mind the subjective significance of privacy. Although the potential consequences of breaches—and sometimes protection—of confidentiality of sensitive information may be severe, policy might be best informed by constant attention to the normative foundation for protection of privacy: the preservation of personal boundaries and, thus, the protection of personal dignity. It is easy to become caught in a cost–benefit analysis that recognizes the sometimes minimal personal *harm* of an intrusion on a client's privacy but minimizes the *wrong* associated with such a violation.

SPECIAL ISSUES RELATED TO CHILDREN'S PRIVACY

Number of Interested Parties

Beyond the "usual" list (for adult clients) of consumers, providers, and third-party payers with an interest in clinical records, the various parties responsible for a child's care (e.g., parents, teachers, child welfare workers) may regard access to confidential information as necessary to fulfill their duties. Accordingly, the legal and practical realities are that children can expect substantially less protection of their personal privacy than can adults. Not only are children subject to nearly round-the-clock surveillance, but also their parents or guardians typically control access to personal information about their children or wards (with some exceptions that will be noted). Even the parents, however, may have other parties looking over their shoulders (into their children's files) without their consent. Through child abuse reporting laws and public health and education statutes, state actors (e.g., public school officials, child welfare authorities) may be able to compel production (as well as release) of information by or about the parents and their care of the children. Thus, for example, the law may require school children to submit to physical examinations and to provide health records. Although the children experience the most direct intrusion (indeed, of bodily privacy), the information that must be disclosed provides evidence of the quality of parental care, and the state is effectively interfering, albeit to a limited degree, in a domain of children's care that parents generally control.

Indeed, it is rare that privacy questions involving children do not implicate the privacy of other individuals and the family as a whole. The diffuse nature of children's personal boundaries is not limited to information about them:

> Consider . . . the KEEP OUT!!! sign on a third grader's bedroom door. The child experiences the room, the possessions in it, and the ideas that they represent or the information that they contain as her own. Her room is the place where the child goes when she "needs some space." In a sense, it defines or, at a minimum, reflects the child's identity. Nonetheless, the child's parents are likely to identify the room and its contents as part of *their* space and to experience an intrusion if a person who is not a member of the family enters it or searches its contents without their permission. In fact, they may regard the child as lacking the competence or the authority to control who enters the room and the level of freedom of exploration that visitors have within it (cf. *United States v. Matlock,* 1974). (Melton, 1991a, p. 66)

The overlap in privacy interests of children, parents, and other caregiving adults is illustrated by the following hypothetical example. On a day early in the school year, Ms. Crump, a public school English teacher, makes a homework assignment: Write an essay describing "How I Spent My Summer Vacation." In effect, Ms. Crump, a representative of the state, is compelling production of information about the children's relationships and their preferences for spending leisure time. It is thus not difficult to imagine some children's resentment of Ms. Crump's implicit demand for information that is "none of her business!"

Parents may be distressed to learn that Johnny and Susie are effectively being required to disclose 1) how they were being shuttled from home to home during the summer as a result of a divorce settlement or 2) why the family was unable to take a vacation this summer (because, for example, Dad was fired from his job or Mom had surgery and treatment for breast cancer). Although the discovery of this family information (some of which certainly could be framed as matters of personal privacy of the parents) is incidental to a task that had a purely instructional purpose, Ms. Crump nonetheless may believe that the parents *should* have disclosed the information—perhaps even that they were *expected* to disclose it—because it may be helpful in understanding Johnny's and Susie's mental health and planning their educational programs. Moreover, others in the school—the guidance counselor, the social worker, the nurse and the psychologist (who may be employees of another agency) in the school health clinic, the retired carpenter who volunteers as a mentor, perhaps even Johnny's football coach and Susie's volleyball coach—may believe that they have a compelling need for such information and thus expect Ms. Crump to disclose it to them. Even if such additional disclosure is not obligatory, Ms. Crump may desire to provide the information to ensure that Johnny and Susie receive help that they may need and, for that matter, that *she* needs to teach them most effectively.

The essay assignment is instructive because that task is not one that most people would regard as particularly sensitive or intrusive. Of course, almost all child mental health services result in elicitation of information that children themselves and their parents and other family members regard as personal and private. Moreover, almost all children who receive mental health services are sometimes under direct or indirect care of adults other than their parents. Teachers, juvenile probation officers, child welfare workers, foster parents, and volunteers may share responsibility for protecting children and enhancing their development.

Need for a Developmental Perspective

As with the interests at stake, the conceptual foundation typically is more complex in questions of children's privacy than in analogous issues pertaining to adults. The nature and salience of children's concerns about privacy and the opportunities for exercising privacy vary as children grow older. Therefore, if proper respect is to be shown in the matters that are most sensitive to children themselves, then a developmental perspective is needed.

The question of children's privacy is "developmental" in another sense. Decisions about whether to disclose mental health information may affect children's educational, career, and other opportunities in adulthood as well as their immediate well-being. At one level, this issue is settled because the Americans with Disabilities Act (ADA) of 1990 (PL 101-336) prohibits discrimination in numerous contexts, including education and employment, on the basis of a record of disability or even the perception of a disability (for the definition of *disability,* see 42 U.S.C. § 12102[2]; for detailed discussion of the ADA and its implications, see Melton, Petrila, Poythress, & Slobogin, 1997, Chapter 13). Therefore, the disclosure of a history of mental disorder in childhood should not by itself narrow the range of opportunities ultimately available.

Such legal protection is effective, however, only when the individual knows that a disclosure has been made, knows that the law offers protection, and asserts the legal protection so that the law can be enforced. If there is a risk that information about childhood diagnosis and treatment is available without the individual's knowledge, then the legal protection against discrimination may be effectively unavailable. Hence, the potential placement of information about a child's mental disorder into a database without the child's or the parents' knowledge is a special case of the general problem of primary concern in this book—the potentially spreading access to mental health information as a result of changes in both information technology (the ease of transfer of information) and the organization of mental health services (the number of people with a possible need to know about the delivery of services). For children, however, this general problem is a reverberating one, with potentially significant effects on movement into higher education and the work force and, therefore, the child's ultimate development into productive adulthood.

The reverberation is not limited to potential consequences in adulthood. Information about children's problems may affect the responses of others in ways that affect the children's development. Consider, for example, a project undertaken by Cadman et al. (1987), in which they conducted a clinical trial of a public health and education program focusing on children registering for kindergarten in three school districts in southern Ontario. Children were randomly assigned to one of three groups: 1) a screening test (the Denver Developmental Screening Test [Frankenburg & Dodds, 1969]), with a community health intervention for the children determined to be at high risk; 2) a screening test, with no special services for the children determined to be at high risk; or 3) no screening test. The intervention for children in the first group was low intensity: referral to the child's physician for an assessment, a review conference between the child's teacher and the school health nurse, parent counseling, and monitoring of the child in school by the school health nurse. When individual academic achievement and cognitive and developmental tests were administered 3 years later, children who had been "screened in" and who had received the community health intervention did not differ from the groups that had received no interventions. However, parents of children who received the intervention had more worry about school progress, and the children who had received the intervention did have more school problems than did the other children.

Because the community intervention in the Cadman et al. study consisted largely of sensitization of parents, health professionals, and teachers to children's developmental risk, that program may have been made to order for self-fulfilling prophecies that might not occur when early intervention programs that are more supportive and better grounded are administered. In that sense, however, the Cadman et al. study is a good analogue to the circumstance that occurs when information about children's problems is divulged on an ad hoc basis (e.g., when a teacher reads a child's file that contains information about mental health problems, and the teacher is not a partner in a specific treatment program for the child).

SCOPE OF PRIVACY INTERESTS

The title of this book (*Privacy **and** Confidentiality in Mental Health Care* [emphasis added]) itself suggests the murkiness of the topic. On the one hand, confidentiality typically is understood as an element of privacy. The retention of intimate information given in confidence shows respect for the individual who divulged the information and enables some measure of preservation of his or her personal boundaries. However, the purposes of confidentiality extend beyond protection of personal privacy. For example, confidentiality may be premised on protection of competitive information ("trade secrets"). Accordingly, health care providers and third-party payers may be increasingly concerned about widespread circulation of information about market demand and service utilization, especially when time and money have been invested in synthesis of such data. What is ironic, therefore, is that providers and payers may sometimes be more directly concerned about the confidentiality of aggregate data than the confidentiality (privacy) of individual records.

There are other purposes of confidentiality that cannot be described as privacy. For example, a hospital may be willing to release information to a researcher who is studying iatrogenic practices only if it may do so in confidence. Although such confidentiality may save hospital administrators from embarrassment and their institutions from lawsuits, it is meaningless to talk about the privacy of the hospital itself; privacy applies to individuals and families, not corporations. However, the pursuit of knowledge about a topic of public importance may require protection of confidentiality. Such a theory underlies the limited privilege of journalists and scholars to shield their sources (see, e.g., *Branzburg v. Hayes,* 1972; *Dow Chemical Co. v. Allen,* 1982; *United States v. Doe,* 1972; for a detailed discussion of the law and ethics of confidentiality in health research, see Gray, Lyons, & Melton, 1995).

On the other hand, privacy clearly extends beyond confidentiality. This general principle applies in mental health services as well as in other contexts. For example, facilities for residential treatment ought to be designed and administered in a manner that permits definition of private spaces; that severely limits searches of residents' person or possessions; that respects modesty in personal hygiene, dress, and sleeping arrangements; and that enables privacy in correspondence, telephone calls, and other communications. That the residents are children does not mean that their privacy interests are unimportant.

Moreover, treatment itself can be evaluated in terms of its intrusiveness (see Melton, Lyons, & Spaulding, 1998). Unfortunately, treatments for children, especially those aimed at children who have conduct disorders or who are in the juvenile justice system, have sometimes been designed to strip away their self-respect as a first step toward resocialization. Measures of such type include degradation rituals (e.g., placing new residents on "level zero") and intense confrontation. Although total institutions, by their nature, are more likely to use highly intrusive procedures (see, e.g., Rivlin & Wolfe, 1985; *State v. Werner,* 1978, p. 913, quoting testimony of R. Hawkins), the key factor is *what* is done, not *where* it is done or *who* does it. Degradation rituals are psychologically intrusive regardless of whether they are performed in a public school, a juvenile justice facility, an outpatient clinic, a group home, or a hospital.

Such highly intrusive procedures should be prohibited as psychologically abusive:

> Laws and agency regulations governing institutional care [and other treatment settings] should go beyond prevention of physical maltreatment. They also must prevent psychological harm and threats to the dignity of the children and youth directly or indirectly under state care. In that regard, institutions and their staff should be barred from interventions designed to humiliate, depersonalize, deprive of outside communication (other than reasonable restrictions on time, place, and manner), isolate (other than brief periods of seclusion when necessary to ensure safety), or otherwise subject youth to significantly greater intrusion upon privacy than expectable in family life.
>
> Neither a therapeutic justification nor consent by a parent or guardian should be a defense to allegations of psychological maltreatment under such a standard, which subsumes only the most egregious assaults upon the personal dignity of children and youth. (Melton & Davidson, 1987, p. 174)

The argument here is principally on deontological grounds. Such dehumanization simply is wrong. However, similar arguments could be made on the basis of clinical considerations. Children's misbehavior sometimes is the product of depression more than of character disorder (Carlson & Cantwell, 1980; Chiles, Miller, & Cox, 1980; Meeks, 1995). In such an instance, a highly intrusive intervention is apt to threaten already fragile self-esteem. By contrast, protection of privacy may enhance self-esteem (Wolfe, 1978). Golan (1978) found, for example, that child psychiatric inpatients living in single bedrooms had significantly higher self-esteem and, unsurprising, significantly more frequent experiences of privacy as chosen aloneness than did inpatients living in multiple-occupancy bedrooms. These differences were observed even though the two groups did not differ in the severity of mental disorder ascribed to them by the program staff.

To summarize, "psychological research and theory on the significance of privacy for the maintenance of self-esteem and development of personal identity is remarkable for its congruence with legal and philosophical discourse on the relation of privacy to human dignity" (Melton, 1991a, pp. 74–75, citing, e.g., Tremper, 1988, and Tremper & Kelly, 1987). Respect for children's dignity is not just the right thing to do; it also promotes children's happiness and development. In that regard, it should come as no surprise that children evaluate the quality of living situations away from their families of origin in large part on the basis of the degree of restriction of liberty and invasion of privacy (Bush, 1980; Rivlin & Wolfe, 1985; Roth & Roth, 1984).

Thus, although this chapter, like the book as a whole, is focused primarily on issues of confidentiality, it is important to remember that the privacy issues in mental health services go beyond protection of the privacy of clinical information (see, e.g., *Milonas v. Williams,* 1982). For example, compelled treatment—the norm in child mental health services, at least from the perspective of the child—not only is restrictive (reducing liberty) but also is intrusive (reducing privacy). Although such intrusions sometimes are justified, clinicians and policy makers should be mindful of their seriousness and should act with due care and minimization of intrusiveness as much as possible.

THE DEVELOPMENTAL PSYCHOLOGY OF PRIVACY

As studied most extensively by Wolfe and her colleagues (Laufer & Wolfe, 1977; Rivlin & Wolfe, 1985; Wolfe, 1978), the experience of privacy is indeed important in the development of children and adolescents. Most fundamental, privacy is significant in the definition of the self in relation to society:

> Through their daily experiences, children and adolescents develop an understanding of the uses and limits of interaction and information management in everyday life. They develop a sense of themselves as separate from and connected to each other, an understanding of the conditions under which to see physical and psychological aloneness or interaction, and understanding of the possible range of such experience and the uses of each of these for self-enhancement or regrouping. At the same time, these experiences give children and adolescents a view of societal norms with respect to certain behaviors and activities and provide a way of interpreting these as valued or not valued, good or bad. In this way, children's experiences with privacy feed back into their sense of self-esteem and help define the range, limits, and consequences of individual autonomy within our society. (Wolfe, 1978, p. 189)

Given privacy's relation to identity formation, it is not surprising that it has particular meaning to adolescents as a marker of self-differentiation and independence (Wolfe, 1978). Relative to younger children, adolescents are especially concerned about privacy of information (distinguished from personal space and bodily privacy); such privacy is probably a prerequisite for development of intimate relationships. Consistent with that developmental trend, self-disclosure is the risk of mental health treatment most often identified by older children and youth, particularly those who have experience in treatment (Kaser-Boyd, Adelman, & Taylor, 1985). Similarly, confidentiality is a common reason for adolescents to seek services from school-based clinics (Palfrey, McGaughey, Cooperman, Fenton, & McManus, 1991).

Hence, the protection of privacy in mental health services is especially important to adolescents. Of course, that conclusion does not imply that the privacy interests of younger children can be ignored. To the contrary, perceptions of privacy reflect the experiences of children of various ages, and privacy is salient even to children in the primary grades. Researchers have assessed the concepts of privacy in children as young as 5 years (Wolfe, 1978). Given that experiences of privacy (aloneness) are seldom volitional for young children, it is not surprising that children do not perceive privacy as the result of an active choice to manage social interaction and information. The relation between experience and perception is also reflected in the fact that control of access to place is especially salient to children in the intermediate grades relative to children in the primary grades (who typically lack such privacy) and adolescents (who feel relatively secure in protection of private places). Attention to such developmental concerns can contribute to a greater sense of self-esteem and personal control.

LEGAL CONTEXT

Whether for ethical or clinical reasons or both, many mental health professionals do wish to respect the privacy of their child clients. Such action is possible, however, only if the law permits it. The following sections examine the legal limits of children's privacy.

Legal Significance of Children's Privacy

Privacy does not appear in the U.S. Constitution but permeates it—a concept that was expressed in the Supreme Court's first case on the constitutional right to privacy in terms of a fit with the "penumbras" of the Constitution (*Griswold v. Connecticut,* 1965). In part because of the difficulty in defining the contours of privacy, the limits of constitutional protection of privacy have been controversial and still in some measure unresolved even for adults. Nonetheless, the Supreme Court has repeatedly recognized the fundamental significance of privacy in the protection of human dignity. For example, in a case that offered the opportunity to overrule *Roe v. Wade* (1973), the Supreme Court instead reaffirmed the importance of privacy in constitutional law:

> Our law affords constitutional protection to personal decisions relating to marriage, procreation, contraception, family relationships, child rearing, and education. Our cases recognize "the right of the individual, married or single, to be free from unwarranted governmental intrusion into matters so fundamentally affecting a person as the decision whether to bear or beget a child." Our precedents "have respected the private realm of family life which the state cannot enter." These matters, involving the most intimate and personal choices a person may make in a lifetime, choices central to personal dignity and autonomy, are central to the liberty protected by the Fourteenth Amendment. At the heart of liberty is the right to define one's own concept of existence, of meaning, of the universe, and of the mastery of human life. Beliefs about these matters could not define the attributes of personhood were they formed under compulsion of the State. (*Planned Parenthood of Southeastern Pennsylvania v. Casey,* 1992, p. 851, citations omitted).[2]

In principle, "intimate and personal choices" are "central to [the] personal dignity and autonomy" of children as well as adults. Although the United States stands alone with Somalia as nonparties to the Convention on the Rights of the Child (1989), that document provides a guidepost. Echoing the core construct in the U.S. Constitution (Tremper, 1988), the Convention focuses on the requisites for *dignity* of children, a concept that is repeatedly, expressly, or implicitly mentioned (Melton, 1991b).

Reflecting the corollary desire of the drafters for an article focusing specifically on the child's right to privacy (Flekkøy & Kaufman, 1997), the Convention on the Rights of the Child established children's right to "protection of the law" against "arbitrary or unlawful interference with his or her privacy, family, home, or correspondence" and "unlawful attacks on his or her honour or reputation" (art. 16). This provision was drawn verbatim from the International Covenant on Civil and Political Rights (1966, art. 17). The intent of the drafters of the Convention on the Rights of the Child as to its scope when applied to children is not clear from the

---

[2]For a more eloquent and expansive—but losing—explication of the personal significance of constitutional protection of privacy, see Justice Blackmun's dissent in *Bowers v. Hardwick* (1986).

travaux (Flekkøy & Kaufman, 1997), but the elements of the article closely match the tort of invasion of privacy as explicated by Warren and Brandeis (1890).

International authority for the significance of a right to privacy in child mental health services can also be found in the Principles for the Protection of Persons with Mental Illness and the Improvement of Mental Health Care (1991). Principle 13(1)(b) of that instrument provides for a right to privacy for all patients in mental health facilities, and Principle 6 specifically recognizes a right to confidentiality of personal information about people with mental illnesses or who are treated as such. These principles flow from the fundamental right to "be treated with humanity and respect for the inherent dignity of the human person" (Principle 1[2]). The principles also demand "special care" in protecting the rights of minors receiving mental health services (Principle 2).

U.S. courts have been more ambivalent about minors' privacy than have the drafters of international human rights treaties. The general trend has been to recognize minors' right to privacy but then to write at length about why it is less important for minors than adults and ultimately to establish a lower standard for abridgement of minors' rights than applies to adults. Thus the Supreme Court has set *significant* rather than *compelling* state interests as the standard for state regulation of adolescents' decisions about abortions (*Planned Parenthood of Central Missouri v. Danforth*, 1976). On the basis of this lower standard of scrutiny, the Supreme Court has permitted states to require notification even of both parents as long as the minor has an opportunity to go before a judge—a mammoth invasion of privacy—and to prove either that she is mature or that an abortion is in her best interests (*Hodgson v. Minnesota*, 1990). The Court has premised this intrusion on "the peculiar vulnerability of children; their inability to make critical decisions in an informed, mature manner; and the importance of the parental role in child rearing" (*Bellotti v. Baird*, 1979, p. 634).

A similar pattern has applied in the Court's cases on privacy in schools under the Fourth Amendment. In *New Jersey v. T.L.O.* (1985), the Court held that it is "indisputable . . . that the Fourteenth Amendment protects the rights of students against encroachment by public school officials" (p. 334), indeed that a search of a student's handbag or person is "undoubtedly a severe violation of subjective expectations of privacy" (p. 338). In drawing that conclusion, the Court recognized that students' handbags often contain "the necessaries of personal hygiene and grooming," as well as "such nondisruptive yet highly personal items as photographs, letters, and diaries" (p. 339).[3]

Nonetheless, the Court upheld the constitutionality of the search by establishing a lower standard (reasonable suspicion) for warrantless searches of school children. In doing so, the Court incredibly found it necessary to contrast the virtual absence of legitimate expectations of privacy in prisons (*Hudson v. Palmer,* 1984): "We are not yet ready to hold that the schools and the prisons need be equated for purposes of the Fourth Amendment" (*New Jersey v. T.L.O.,* 1985, pp. 338–339). Nonetheless, the Court adopted its lower standard by observing that intrusions on students' privacy are commonplace. The logic seemed to be analogous to the Court's earlier holding that preventive detention of juvenile respondents in delinquency proceedings is justifiable because juveniles' interest in liberty "must be qualified by the recognition that juveniles, unlike adults, are always in some form of custody" (*Schall v. Martin,* 1984, p. 265). The practical import of the cavalier minimization of privacy interests was demonstrated by the subsequent application of *New Jersey v. T.L.O.* by at least one federal circuit court to uphold a warrantless strip search by a vice principal (*Williams ex rel. Williams v. Ellington,* 1991).

Subsequently, the Supreme Court has applied *New Jersey v. T.L.O.* to hold that blanket drug tests of high school athletes are permitted under the Fourth Amendment (*Vernonia School District 47J v. Acton,* 1995). In reaching that judgment, the Court said that the critical fact in the case was that "the subjects of the [Student Athlete Drug] Policy are 1) children, who 2) have been committed to the temporary custody of the state as schoolmaster" (p. 2391). The Court did note that the requirement to provide disclosure of medications that a student was taking prior to the drug screen "raises some cause for concern" (imagine, e.g., a student being required to reveal that he or she is taking psychotropic medication), but the Court concluded that "the invasion of privacy was not significant" (p. 2394).

---

[3]An interesting and unresolved gender discrimination issue applies here. *New Jersey v. T.L.O.* (1985) involved a school official's search of a teenage girl's handbag to determine whether cigarettes (possession of which would have been a violation of school rules) were present. Suppose that the assistant principal had instead thrust his hand into a teenage boy's front pants pocket. This hypothetical situation illustrates the importance of considering the meaning of a search or other intrusion on privacy from the child's perspective.

Ambiguity of Legal Protection of Children's Privacy

Of course, decision making about release of clinical information generally is based on prevailing state law, not federal constitutional doctrines. Unfortunately, the relevant law is often murky and confusing.

The general principle is that parents have the authority to make decisions about their children's treatment, including release of information. When one or both parents have surrendered custody, whether voluntarily or involuntarily, the legal guardian will ordinarily have authority to make decisions regarding health care. A separation or divorce settlement will specify the parent(s) who retain legal custody. A parent lacking physical custody may still share in joint legal custody; providers should clarify the custody arrangement in determining who may make decisions about a child's treatment. When a court has taken control of a child because of maltreatment or delinquency, legal as well as physical custody typically will be vested in the state. In such an instance, it is common for a public employee (usually a state social worker) to serve as the child's legal guardian (not to be confused with a guardian *ad litem*—an individual who represents a child's interests in litigation).

A voluntary transfer of physical custody for the purpose of treatment (e.g., admission to a residential treatment center) need not and indeed should not require parents to relinquish legal custody to the state. Without such surrender, parents retain control over release of information about their children. However, a *de facto* requirement of surrender of legal custody to obtain financing of treatment sometimes occurs in the majority of states (Cohen et al., 1993). The Second Circuit Court of Appeals has held that such a requirement does not violate federal law (*Joyner v. Dumpson,* 1983).

Notwithstanding the general authority of parents, a "mature minor" rule has applied in the common law. Under that rule, health professionals are free from liability for treating older minors who understand the nature and potential consequences of treatment and who consent independently to it (Wadlington, 1983). Some states (e.g., Arkansas [Ark. Code Ann. §20-9-602 (Supp. 1995)]; Mississippi [Miss. Code Ann. §41-41-3 (1993)]) have codified the mature minor rule, and others (e.g., Virginia [Va. Code Ann. §54.1-2969 (Michie 1994)]) have appeared to provide an unlimited right of children to consent to mental health or substance abuse services. Because of the common-law requirement of informed consent, the latter statutes may in fact embody a mature minor rule even though no such standard appears in the relevant statutory code. Still other states have provided minors above a certain age (e.g., 14 in Alabama

[Ala. Code §§22-8-3–22-8-4 (1990)]) but below the ordinary age of majority to consent to treatment independently. In addition to mature minor rules, states often permit independent consent by minors to treatment when they are emancipated through financial independence or marriage (e.g., California [Cal. Fam. Code §§7001–7002, 7050–7051, 7110, 7120–7122 (West 1994)]) or when the provider believes that delaying services to obtain parental consent (including instances in which the minor is denying access to the parents) will result in harm to the minor's health (e.g., Minnesota [Minn. Stat. Ann. §§144.341–144.347 (West 1989)]).

Unfortunately, even when the state statutes provide a clear rule for consent to treatment, they rarely indicate expressly whether the authority to consent to treatment is accompanied by the authority to consent to release of information or to withhold information from parents.[4] The answer should depend on the theory underlying the consent statute. If, on the one hand, it were intended to recognize minors' privacy in a particularly sensitive domain, then the authority to consent to treatment probably implies control over the resulting information. If, on the other hand, the primary motive of legislatures or courts providing independent access to treatment for mature minors was to ensure that troubled children who might be deterred from treatment by a requirement of parental consent do receive services, then there still may be a desire at least to inform parents about their children's problems and any help that they are receiving. Parents, then, could monitor the quality of services and become a partner in treatment.

The Juvenile Justice Standards (Institute of Judicial Administration/American Bar Association Juvenile Justice Standards Project, 1980, Standards 4.2, 4.3, 4.7, & 4.9) provided an interesting attempt to accommodate these interests. Under the standards, minors age 14 or older would be able to consent independently to mental health services, but they could do so for only three sessions without

---

[4]Such statutes are often also silent on the questions of whether children may refuse services to which their parents have consented and, regardless, whether parents control the information when they are the consenting party.

Even when the law is clear on the myriad of issues relating to the limits of children's autonomy and privacy, however, the law on the books will make little difference if state agencies and professional associations make no effort to inform practitioners, if the practitioners make no effort to inform children and parents, or if the practitioners decide to pursue other practices regardless of the law. (See Melton, 1981, for a study showing minimal knowledge and impact of a statutory reform to increase children's independent access to mental health services.)

their parents' being notified. By contrast, minors of any age could consent independently to substance abuse treatment with notification of the parents only if the minor did not object or the clinician determined that failing to notify the parents would seriously endanger the minor's health. In the latter instance, the clinician would be able to inform a parent without the minor's consent "only after making all reasonable efforts to persuade the minor to consent to notification of the parent" (Standard 4.2[B][2][b]). Minors who did consent independently to treatment would assume financial responsibility, but confidentiality might be preserved by a requirement that their insurers pay the bills in such instances without informing the policy holders.[5]

PRINCIPLES FOR PUBLIC POLICY

Recognizing Zones of Privacy

The most fundamental principle ought to be that children's privacy in mental health services is recognized as a fundamental interest. Accordingly, children should be able not only to consent independently to mental health services but also to control the release of information under such circumstances. Even when parents do control the information, children ought to be able to reserve some intimate details—in effect, a zone of privacy—that are not disclosed to responsible adults except when serious danger would otherwise result.

Nonetheless, as discussed in the conclusion to this chapter, the general norm ought to be *shared* decision making. It is possible to accommodate the interests of both children and parents so that some measure of privacy for both children and parents is retained without compromising the parents' ability to care for their children.

Relation Between Security and Sensitivity of Information

The principle that should guide the definition of zones of privacy is that the more sensitive the information is—that is, the more that its release would be viewed as a personal violation exposing the subject of the information[6] to degradation, embarrassment, or stigma—

---

[5]An example of a particularly muddled statute on minors' consent is Nebraska's (Neb. Rev. Stat. §71-504 [1996]), which provides for independent and confidential consent by minors to diagnosis and treatment of sexually transmitted diseases but then makes parents financially responsible for the services. Presumably, this statute could be fully implemented only if parents received a bill for unknown services provided to an unknown individual for an unknown condition!

[6]Note that this criterion is not necessarily defined by the identity of the individual in whose record information is stored or who serves as the

(continued)

the stronger should be its protection. This principle should affect not only the definition of domains in which children have ultimate control over information about them but also the general practices about information sharing.

School-based mental health services provide a good example. A rule of reason has become the conventional practice in regard to access to information in school-based mental health services (Dryfoos, 1994). To infuse a mental health perspective into the schools (e.g., to permit ongoing consultation to teachers and other school personnel), mental health professionals who are based in the schools should have access to information about children's school performance, even when the children are not clients of the mental health program. Otherwise, an artificial and maladaptive barrier is erected, and it interferes with the school's own work because the mental health professionals—even if employed by other agencies—ought to be seen as part of the school staff. For the purpose of access to school records (and most other purposes), school-based clinicians should be viewed as agents of the schools with routine-use access to educational information.

At the same time, teachers cannot reasonably be viewed as part of the mental health center staff; they are not "mental-health-center-based teachers." Moreover, there are few circumstances in which detailed mental health information—often the most private thoughts of children and other family members—is necessary for educational planning. Therefore, teachers should not have routine-use access to the clinical records maintained by the school-based mental health professionals. Informed consent by responsible parties to release the information should be necessary before it is disclosed to school personnel. (As noted previously, it is desirable that such consent procedures go beyond current legally required practices to enable shared decision making with due deference to children's personal privacy interests.) Even in that context, clinicians should limit the information to that for which there is a legitimate use by school personnel, and they should be careful to provide appropriate explanations and cautions about personal information that may be especially sensitive or prone to misinterpretation.

---

source of the information. As noted previously in this chapter, mental health information about children almost always may be subsumed within zones of privacy for other people, particularly their parents. Therefore, the willingness of children themselves to provide broad access to personal information does not resolve the issue, even in instances in which the law does recognize their self-determination in decisions about the release of personal information.

Need for Standardization

On a day-to-day basis, much of the concern about confidentiality laws and policies as an undue barrier to coordination and integration of services emanates from uncertainties created by seemingly arbitrary variations in policies and conventional practices. In an effort to reduce these variations without reducing protection of privacy, Soler, Shotton, and Bell recommended that the federal government establish "a consistent set of requirements for written releases of confidential information. . ., a basic set of circumstances in which information may be shared without consent," and "a model interagency agreement for information sharing for the purpose of improving service delivery" (1993, pp. 47–48). Such consistent policies and procedures would go far toward elimination of confidentiality as an excuse or simply a perceived barrier to implementation of flexible, individualized services.

Soler et al.'s recommendations were derived from their study of confidentiality-related statutes, regulations, and practices in California, Iowa, New York, Washington State, and the federal government:

> From this analysis, the authors reached a clear conclusion: Confidentiality provisions are not significant barriers to interagency collaboration, and virtually all information-sharing problems can be resolved by using mechanisms such as written releases that are authorized by statutes and regulations. Nevertheless, the study demonstrated the need to demystify "confidentiality" as a barrier to interagency efforts by discussing and organizing the issues in a clear, straightforward manner. Many agency personnel feel that confidentiality of records is a highly technical issue, largely inaccessible to non-lawyers, shrouded in secrecy and impenetrable. That is not true. The most experienced agency administrators were virtually unanimous in their belief that confidentiality issues are frequently overblown and often cover up underlying interagency conflicts over turf, "ownership" of the data, and budget control. The agency administrators agreed with the authors of this study that confidentiality issues are eminently resolvable by the agencies and clients affected. (1993, p. 3)

Soler et al. identified a myriad of techniques to avoid artificial barriers between agencies attempting to integrate their services on behalf of individual children or classes of children. Soler et al.'s book includes examples of illustrative statutes, regulations, interagency agreements, and standing court orders. Such existing instruments may serve as the foundation for newly standardized approaches to client confidentiality, particularly when it is being used as a barrier to more responsive services.

Need to Limit Access to Sensitive Information

In some circumstances, there may be insufficient protection of privacy. The problem described as "reverberation" of disclosure of personal information is illustrative. In this regard, the consequences for children may be especially profound because personal information may be used to limit opportunities for entry into a place in the community (higher education or a job). This constriction of opportunities may occur directly through discrimination or indirectly through self-fulfilling prophecies.

The problem of direct effects is a special case of the general issues about databases, as addressed by Petrila and others in this book. Such misuse often is illegal under the ADA, but enforcement of the law is difficult because consumers often are unaware when health information is disclosed. In that regard, the Clinton administration's proposal (Shalala, 1997) to provide health care consumers with access to information about requests for health records may be an important step. Indeed, one can make a case that the step should be bigger: that consumers be provided not just with access but instead with notice when clinical information is being released to a third party.

The problem of indirect effects may be reduced by development of professional norms limiting routine-use access to personal information that may be prone to misinterpretation and that is unlikely to be useful by particular classes of people who may ordinarily have access in current practice. In that regard, as the sensitivity of information increases, so should the security of that information increase. To return to the example given in that discussion, school teachers simply do not have a legitimate need for detailed mental health information. Even if the need may be legitimate, the risk of misinterpretation is too great to permit access to the information without an accompanying explanation of its meaning.

From a more general perspective, education in the various professions serving children probably should have a greater emphasis on the (in)validity of much personal information that is commonly recorded but that offers little for short-term treatment planning or long-term prediction of children's well-being. The problem of who has access to personal information about children is apt to become more significant as the organization of services (often already including numerous agencies, each with its own routine uses and third-party payers, managers, and auditors) becomes increasingly complex. This issue would be less acute if information of dubious utility simply were not recorded.

A DILEMMA AND A PARTIAL SOLUTION

Underlying much of the debate about the limits of privacy for minors, especially adolescents, is a dilemma. On the one hand, affording to adolescents control over their personal information

> Denotes respect for the dignity and personhood of the adolescent; it provides the opportunity for the development of intimate relationships and recognition that the adolescent now faces decisions which in our culture are marked as "private" and belonging to the individual. (Melton, 1983, pp. 488–489)

On the other hand, protection of their informational privacy sometimes shields adolescents from scrutiny of illicit behavior. In fact, situations in which adolescents report having difficulty in managing personal information typically relate to "deviant" activities such as sexual involvement and substance use (Wolfe, 1978).

Of course, the risk that protection of privacy sometimes will interfere with the administration of justice is not limited to adolescents. In applying the Fourth Amendment, society recognizes that the guilty sometimes will avoid justice, but we are prepared to suffer that cost to protect individual and family privacy. No one wants to live in a society in which, for example, random or blanket searches are the order of the day, even though such a society might have much less crime than we experience today.

In the case of children and adolescents, however, there is limited legal recognition of autonomy, and many adults (especially parents but also teachers, principals, foster parents, child welfare workers, etc.) share responsibility for their protection. Consequently, many adults believe that they have a need to know about the details of children's experiences. As noted previously, there are many circumstances in which various adults do have a legal right of access to information about children, although there also are some situations in which even parents ordinarily cannot intrude on their children's privacy and others in which parents' and children's interests in regard to confidentiality may be adverse (e.g., when abuse is alleged).

Even in the circumstances in which children can consent to treatment independently and confidentially, it is probable that confidentiality is more limited than for adult clients:

> Although there is no . . . duty to warn the family of an adult client's suicidal tendencies (*Bellah v. Greenson,* 1978), the fact that both the parents and the state are legally obligated to protect dependent minors

> from harm might constitute sufficient reason to impose such a duty
> when the therapist is treating a minor. In fact, it could be argued that
> the parents' duty to care for and control their children entitles them to
> be informed of self-destructive or violent behavior that does not reach
> suicidal or homicidal proportions. There is, however, little case law on
> this question. Therefore, the clinician is well advised to establish a pol-
> icy regarding disclosures to parents, discuss that policy with clients
> when beginning treatment, and carefully document both the policy it-
> self and the reasons for any exceptions made to it. (Melton & Ehren-
> reich, 1992, p. 1046)

Although children's privacy may be limited in practice, parents' and children's interests in the confidentiality of clinical data
are often similar or at least compatible. On the one hand, parents
and children generally share an interest in protecting the family
from embarrassment (see *Merriken v. Cressman,* 1973). On the other
hand, family members often share interests in securing services and
enhancing the accuracy of assessments. Moreover, parents typically
recognize the need for children to have some measure of privacy,
both as a matter of ethics (mutual respect) and as a contributor to
the efficacy of services. Conversely, children typically recognize
parents' special roles in their lives, including the parents' involvement in obtaining and monitoring services for the family. Both parents and school-age children typically can appreciate the unfairness
of either parents' or children's disclosing information that one party
or the other regards as highly private without at least so informing
them.

Accordingly, the foundation is commonly present for *shared*
decision making about disclosure of clinical information concerning children and their families. Such an approach is consistent with
the Convention on the Rights of the Child (1989, article 12), which
requires parties to "assure to the child who is capable of forming his
or her own views the right to express those views freely in all matters affecting the child, the view of the child being given due weight
in accordance with the age and maturity of the child." Note that this
standard, which regulates state (not parental) behavior (thus, e.g.,
the conduct of a publicly supported health professional seeking
consent for treatment of the child), entitles the child not to *self-
determination* but instead to *participation.* Note further that this
right accrues when the child is quite young (when the child is old
enough to state a preference).

Following such a framework, the clinician should negotiate the
limits of privacy. In most circumstances, both the parents and the
child should be informed about requests to share or seek personal

information. Although the parents may have the ultimate legal authority to give or deny consent, the clinician can establish a norm of consultation so that the child has an opportunity to have a say before a decision is made. Similarly, the parents (or the child in instances in which the child has decision-making authority) may partially waive their right of access so that the child (or the parents) retains most control over particular kinds of information; certain exceptions may be agreed on in advance. For example, school-based health clinics often ask parents to waive their right to obtain information except in limited dangerous situations (Gelfman & Schwab, 1991). Such negotiated protection of confidentiality may be jeopardized as school-based clinics increasingly turn to conventional sources of health care financing and both payers and policy holders are informed about children's evaluation and treatment (Palfrey et al., 1991).

CONCLUSION

Although real quandaries involving genuine conflicts of interests do occur, the fact that privacy rights typically can be waived leaves the door open for negotiation of arrangements in which the various interests can be accommodated. Such a process could provide a model for mutually respectful resolution of family conflicts. It also could provide a model for resolution of conflicts between, on the one side, parties outside the family and, on the other side, the whole family or individual family members. In short, although problems of privacy, especially those involving children, are difficult, they typically are tractable when a humane approach is taken to identification and accommodation of the interests at stake.

REFERENCES

Americans with Disabilities Act (ADA) of 1990, PL 101-336, 42 U.S.C. §§ 12101 *et seq.*

Bellotti v. Baird, 443 U.S. 622 (1979).

Bowers v. Hardwick, 478 U.S. 186 (1986).

Branzburg v. Hayes, 408 U.S. 665 (1972).

Bush, M. (1980). Institutions for dependent and neglected children: Therapeutic option of choice or last resort? *American Journal of Orthopsychiatry, 50,* 239–255.

Cadman, D., Chambers, L.W., Walter, S.D., Ferguson, R., Johnston, N., & McNamee, J. (1987). Evaluation of public health preschool child developmental screening: The process and outcomes of a community program. *American Journal of Public Health, 77,* 45–51.

Carlson, G.A., & Cantwell, D.P. (1980). Unmasking masked depression in children and adolescents. *American Journal of Psychiatry, 137,* 445–449.

Chiles, J.A., Miller, M.L., & Cox, G.B. (1980). Depression in an adolescent delinquent population. *Archives of General Psychiatry, 37,* 1179–1184.

Cohen, R., Preiser, L., Gottlieb, S., Harris, R., Baker, J., & Sonenklar, N. (1993). Relinquishing custody as a requisite for receiving services for children with serious emotional disorders: A review. *Law and Human Behavior, 17,* 121–134.

Convention on the Rights of the Child, U.N. Doc. A/Res/44/25 (1989).

Dow Chemical Co. v. Allen, 672 F.2d 1262 (7th Cir. 1982).

Dryfoos, J.G. (1994). *Full-service schools: A revolution in health and social services for children, youth, and families.* San Francisco: Jossey-Bass.

Flekkøy, M.G., & Kaufman, N.H. (1997). *The participation rights of the child: Rights and responsibilities in family and society.* London: Kingsley.

Frankenburg, W.K., & Dodds, J.B. (1969). *The Denver Developmental Screening Test.* Denver: University of Colorado Medical Center.

Gelfman, M.H.B., & Schwab, N.C. (1991). School health services and educational records: Conflicts in the law. *Education Law Reporter, 64,* 319–338.

Golan, M.B. (1978). Privacy, interaction, and self-esteem. Unpublished doctoral dissertation, City University of New York.

Gray, J.N., Lyons, P.M., Jr., & Melton, G.B. (1995). *Ethical and legal issues in AIDS research.* Baltimore: Johns Hopkins University Press.

Griswold v. Connecticut, 381 U.S. 479 (1965).

Hodgson v. Minnesota, 497 U.S. 417 (1990).

Hudson v. Palmer, 468 U.S. 576 (1984).

Institute of Judicial Administration/American Bar Association Juvenile Justice Standards Project. (1980). *Juvenile Justice Standards: Standards relating to rights of minors.* Cambridge, MA: Ballinger.

International Covenant on Civil and Political Rights, U.N. Doc. A/Res/ 21/2200 (1966).

Joyner v. Dumpson, 712 F.2d 770 (2d Cir. 1983).

Kaser-Boyd, N., Adelman, H.S., & Taylor, L. (1985). Minors' ability to identify risks and benefits of therapy. *Professional Psychology: Research and Practice, 16,* 411–417.

Laufer, R.S., & Wolfe, M. (1977). Privacy as a concept and a social issue: A multidimensional developmental theory. *Journal of Social Issues, 33*(3), 22–42.

Meeks, J.E. (1995). Hospitalization and inpatient treatment. In G.P. Sholevar (Ed.), *Conduct disorders in children and adolescents* (pp. 299–317). Washington, DC: American Psychiatric Press.

Melton, G.B. (1981). Effects of a state law permitting minors to consent to psychotherapy. *Professional Psychology, 12,* 647–654.

Melton, G.B. (1983). Minors and privacy: Are legal and psychological concepts compatible? *Nebraska Law Review, 62,* 455–493.

Melton, G.B. (1991a). Respecting boundaries: Minors, privacy, and behavioral research. In B. Stanley & J. Sieber (Eds.), *Social research on children and adolescents: Ethical issues* (pp. 65–84). Thousand Oaks, CA: Sage Publications.

Melton, G.B. (1991b). Socialization in the global community: Respect for the dignity of children. *American Psychologist, 46,* 66–71.

Melton, G.B., & Davidson, H.A. (1987). Child protection and society: When should the state intervene? *American Psychologist, 42,* 172–175.

Melton, G.B., & Ehrenreich, N.S. (1992). Ethical and legal issues in mental health services for children. In C.E. Walker & M.C. Roberts (Eds.), *Handbook of clinical child psychology* (2nd ed., pp. 1035–1055). New York: John Wiley & Sons.

Melton, G.B., Lyons, P.M., Jr., & Spaulding, W.J. (1998). *No place to go: Civil commitment of minors.* Lincoln: University of Nebraska Press.

Melton, G.B., Petrila, J., Poythress, N.G., & Slobogin, C. (1997). *Psychological evaluations for the courts: A handbook for mental health professionals and lawyers* (2nd ed.). New York: Guilford Press.

Merriken v. Cressman, 364 F. Supp. 913 (E.D. Pa. 1973).

Milonas v. Williams, 691 F.2d 931 (10th Cir. 1982).

New Jersey v. T.L.O., 469 U.S. 325 (1985).

Olmstead v. United States, 277 U.S. 438 (1928).

Palfrey, J.S., McGaughey, M.J., Cooperman, P.J., Fenton, T., & McManus, M.A. (1991). Financing health services in school-based clinics: Do nontraditional programs tap traditional funding sources? *Journal of Adolescent Health, 12,* 233–239.

Planned Parenthood of Central Missouri v. Danforth, 428 U.S. 52 (1976).

Planned Parenthood of Southeastern Pennsylvania v. Casey, 505 U.S. 833 (1992).

Principles for the Protection of Persons with Mental Illness and the Improvement of Mental Health Care, U.N. Doc. A/Res/46/119 (1991).

Roe v. Wade, 410 U.S. 113 (1973).

Rivlin, L.G., & Wolfe, M. (1985). *Institutional settings in children's lives.* New York: John Wiley & Sons.

Roth, E.A., & Roth, L.H. (1984, April). *Children's feelings about psychiatric hospitalization: Legal and ethical implications.* Paper presented at the meeting of the American Orthopsychiatric Association, Toronto, Ontario, Canada.

Schall v. Martin, 467 U.S. 253 (1984).

Shalala, D. (1997, July). *Protecting privacy of health information.* Speech to the National Press Club, Washington, D.C.

Soler, M.I., Shotton, A.C., & Bell, J.R. (1993). *Glass walls: Confidentiality provisions and interagency collaborations.* San Francisco: Youth Law Center.

State v. Werner, 242 S.E. 2d 907 (W.Va. 1978).

Tremper, C.R. (1988). Respect for the human dignity of minors: What the Constitution requires. *Syracuse Law Review, 39,* 1293–1349.

Tremper, C.R., & Kelly, M.P. (1987). The mental health rationale for policies fostering minors' autonomy. *International Journal of Law and Psychiatry, 10,* 111–127.

United States v. Doe, 460 F.2d 328 (1st Cir. 1972).

United States v. Matlock, 415 U.S. 164 (1974).

Vernonia School District 47J v. Acton, 115 S.Ct. 2386 (1995).

Wadlington, W.J. (1983). Consent to medical care for minors: The legal framework. In G.B. Melton, G.P. Koocher, & M.J. Saks (Eds.), *Children's competence to consent* (pp. 57–74). New York: Plenum.

Warren, S., & Brandeis, L. (1890). The right to privacy. *Harvard Law Review, 4,* 193–220.

Williams *ex rel.* Williams v. Ellington, 936 F.2d 881 (6th Cir. 1991).

Wolfe, M. (1978). Childhood and privacy. In I. Altman & J. Wohlwill (Eds.), *Human behavior and environment: Advances in theory and research* (Vol. 3, pp. 175–222). New York: Plenum.

5

Clinical Issues in Mental Health Care

Marcia Kraft Goin

As battles for access are waged *outside* the clinician's office by those who believe that they can benefit by learning what has gone on *inside* the office, the clinician faces the daunting task of balancing the need to know with the need to protect. The importance of privacy and trust as principles of the doctor–patient relationship is deeply rooted in medical practice and can be found within the fundamental tenets of the Hippocratic Oath: "All that may come to my knowledge in the exercise of my profession or in daily commerce with men which ought not to be spread abroad, I will keep secret and will never reveal."

People seek medical care when they are suffering, both mentally and physically. In this state of vulnerability, they often pour out their hearts, telling life stories that they believe will be kept in confidence. This storytelling is important for the therapeutic process, especially in psychiatric practice. It is through these tales of frightening symptoms, excesses, indiscretions, violence, and family illnesses that the clinician is provided with the necessary details to make an informed diagnosis and treatment plan.

In a time of crisis, people often will drop their natural reserve and answer any and all questions in their quest for relief from their pain and suffering. As patients recover from the severe pain of a heart attack or the fear induced by a panic attack, the inhibitions and constraints return. A despairing adolescent, flooded with anxiety and depression, brought to the emergency room after she slashes her wrists is likely, at the height of this emotional crisis, to reveal a great deal about herself to an understanding physician. This leaves behind a record of personally sensitive information that, under different circumstances, the patient would never consider revealing and never believed would be disclosed. Similarly, a patient vomiting blood will readily tell at least 50% of the truth about his alcohol intake. At another time, it may take a special confidence in the physician to enable the patient to get past shame and denial and tell the whole truth. Clinicians should have a strong sense of responsibility to protect vulnerable patients. Clinicians also need a sensitive appreciation of the need for confidentiality if a trusting doctor–patient relationship is to develop and survive.

Several factors endanger the privacy that has been an expectable part of the doctor–patient relationship. While the 20th century has seen a quantum leap forward in medical technology, there has been a concurrent escalation in cost as traditional tools such as the stethoscope have been forsaken for the diagnostic prowess and technical wizardry of high-priced computerized axial tomography (CAT) scans and magnetic resonance imaging (MRI) scans. Along with the escalating costs attendant to providing the latest in medical advances, an entire health industry devoted solely to the issue of cost containment has developed. Managed medical care necessarily revolves around concepts such as service rationing, limiting access to expensive care, and overseeing those contracted to provide such care. Third-party payers and their managers have turned an intense spotlight on the activities of health care professions, hospitals and clinics, and, last, the health record itself in an attempt to ensure financial accountability. It is the belief of payers and managers that unhindered access to any and all sources of information related to a patient's health is necessary for the performance of their functions.

At the same time, health care professionals and patients' rights advocates are waging an ongoing battle to protect the confidentiality of patients' health information and preserve the climate of trust necessary for optimal patient care. Confidentiality is highlighted as a core responsibility in the Code of Ethics of all of the professional mental health organizations. The willingness to seek treatment and the ability to speak openly with one's health care professional are inextricably intertwined with concerns about trust and the eroding of privacy of medical information. Numerous cases of unauthorized disclosures demonstrate the negative consequences of failures to provide confidentiality and the misuse of medical information. The provision of mental health services is particularly affected by the erosion of privacy rights. Because of the unfortunate stigma associated with mental illness and embarrassment about discussing problems, the added concerns over confidentiality intensify the already present reluctance of individuals to seek treatment.

There are times when maintaining the safety of the public and/or of the patient outweighs the need to maintain confidentiality. The assessment of such risk requires vigilance and thoughtful evaluation. In most cases, however, the health care professional must struggle to find ways to keep silent. To do otherwise can cause the patient personal damage, affect self-esteem, disrupt relationships, and destroy needed trust. The Seventh Circuit Court stated in reviewing the case of *Jaffee v. Redmond,* "The patient's ability to communicate freely without fear of public disclosure is the key to successful therapy."

TREATMENT-RELATED PRIVACY CONCERNS OF ADULTS

The stigma of mental illness looms large in people's minds. Despite constant educational efforts on the part of both professionals and lay groups, it is difficult to reverse the spontaneous negative public reaction when it is discovered that someone is receiving mental health treatment. Be it a politician, lawyer, next-door neighbor, or future son-in-law, an alarm goes off upon hearing, "He's in psychiatric treatment."

At the Los Angeles County–USC Psychiatric Outpatient Clinic, a special treatment program was designed for depressed and economically deprived mothers of preschool children. The innovative treatment approach utilized the unique skills of a social worker who had worked with delinquent girls and their young children in a backyard nursery school. Engaging the mothers and their children in a program of parallel play helped these mothers to improve their parenting capabilities while also receiving psychological guidance. The plan at the Los Angeles County–USC Psychiatric Outpatient Clinic was to organize a similar program for depressed women with preschool children, anticipating that the setting and the psychological interventions would be therapeutic.

In search of women in need, the clinicians met with the leaders of a local Head Start program located in one of Los Angeles' economically disadvantaged sections. The leaders were enthusiastic about the project and quickly identified 10 women who they believed would benefit from the proposed treatment program. These women were obviously struggling with symptoms of depression.

The program was a great idea, but it never happened! Only one of the women agreed to come to the clinic. The others were afraid to register; without their registering, the clinic could not legally provide the service. What were they afraid of? First was the social stigma. Second was the fear that participation would affect their welfare benefits. Third was the pervasive distrust and uneasiness about privacy and the fate of their records within the county system.

This underscores what is common knowledge: There are large numbers of people who *never* seek treatment because they fear exposure. The knowledge and encouragement about the benefits of the program were not enough to outweigh the women's fear of information leakage in the system.

The exposure that poor patients in the public sector have experienced for years is now spreading throughout all strata of society. Increasing enrollment in managed care programs, the computerization of records, utilization reviews, and efforts to increase efficiency and control costs make the potential for exposure a common reality.

In the private sector, corporate employees at all levels are increasingly concerned about potential breaches of confidentiality and the consequent detrimental effect on their employability, promotions, job security, health and life insurance premiums, and future custody issues. These matters greatly trouble prospective patients, and anecdote after anecdote confirms their worst fears:

- According to Aetna, one company carrying their insurance requested identifiable medical information on its employees so it could fire an employee with AIDS ("What to Watch for in Health Care Reform," 1994).
- A man's admission to his doctor of youthful experimentation with marijuana was entered into his computerized records and later used as an excuse by his insurance company for denying him medical benefits ("On-line Medical Records Raise Privacy Fears," 1995).

As the abuses of medical records multiply and the planned computerization of medical information becomes a reality, there will be a profound impact on a public that is already reluctant to pursue mental health treatment. Lindethal and Thomas (1982) asked nonpsychiatric and psychiatric patients about their privacy concerns. Among the nonpsychiatric patients, 33% said that the possible loss of privacy would, at least to *some extent,* deter them from seeking therapy. Of the psychiatric patients, 22% reported that they had *held back* from seeking psychotherapy because of fears of disclosure, and 45% continued to be concerned about this possibility.

The public's fear that they will be harmed by exposure of their medical information has been underscored by the pressure in many states, as well as in the 104th Congress, to enact legislation that will protect the privacy of genetic information. Scientific advances have made the mapping and sequencing of the entire human genome an exciting and amazing medical advance. The ability to do genetic screening and the possibilities of gene therapy potentially touch the lives of everyone. The positive aspects of this medical advance are coupled with the risk of discrimination by the release of predictive and presymptomatic genetic test results to employers, insurers, and others. Concern about the risk has resulted in a flurry of activity to try to maintain the confidentiality of such information. The Human Genome Project speaks to everyone, and everyone should understand that it is this type of vulnerability that each person feels when he or she decides to make a call to a mental health professional (McLean, 1994; Melhman, Kodish, Whitehouse, Zinn, & Sollitto, 1996; Rothstein, 1995; Shore, Berg, Wynne, & Folstein, 1993).

TREATMENT-RELATED PRIVACY CONCERNS OF CHILDREN AND ADOLESCENTS

Unlike adolescents or adults who are seeking treatment for themselves, parents who seek treatment for their children are often hindered more by a sense of failure and embarrassment than by fear of stigmatizing their child. Anxious about their parenting skills, they fear that some failure on their part has caused the problem. It is important for the clinician to recognize the potential danger of the paper trail that begins with that first visit. This information, if uncontrolled, can affect future acceptance to schools of choice, as well as job options and health and life insurance.

The Institute of Medicine has advocated the adoption of computer-based patient records as standard medical practice in the United States (Woodard, 1995). Were this proposal to be implemented, it would generate a computer-based, continuous chronological history of a patient's medical care. Furthermore, this initiative would lead to the establishment of a national health care data network that would record every medical encounter in the United States. The clinician treating a child is torn between considerations of efficiency and research and the potentially devastating consequences on the child's future if indiscretions occur.

As children grow into adolescents, the efforts of therapeutic work shift from a family setting to direct engagement with the adolescent. Numerous studies (e.g., Cheng, Savageau, Sattler, & DeWitt, 1993; Ford, Millstein, Halpern-Feisher, & Irwin, 1997; Ginsberg et al., 1995) have shown that confidentiality is a major factor in overcoming adolescents' reluctance to seek treatment. Ford et al. (1997), in a randomized study of 562 high school students, learned that concerns about privacy in clinical settings decreased the students' willingness to seek health care for sensitive problems and that when they do go, their concerns may inhibit their communication with physicians. Although adolescents expect confidentiality and privacy, Cheng et al. (1993) found that adolescents' distrust of the system is high. In a survey of 1,295 students in 9th–12th grade, 86% reported they would go to their regular physician for a physical illness whereas only 57% would go there for questions about pregnancy, AIDS, or substance abuse (Ginsberg et al., 1995). The latter were issues that they wished to keep private.

The adolescents' responses are not surprising given the developmental issues with which adolescents struggle during that period of their life. Engaged in the process of mastering separation, individuation, and eventual autonomy, "adolescent rebellion," distrust of adults, and turning to peers for identification and support are common occurrences. There is a natural assumption that the adults in their world will not understand them and certainly will not approve of the many internal and external struggles with which they must contend.

Ginsberg et al. (1995) emphasized that adolescents are active participants in the decision to seek health care for themselves. Those who design systems to meet the needs of adolescents must understand and address their special concerns.

FEAR OF DISCLOSURE AND THE RETREAT FROM THERAPY

Although privacy laws have been enacted since the 1960s (e.g., in a study of 108 nonpatients, 42% reported that they would be less likely to be open in therapy if their communications were not absolutely protected), this issue is still of great concern to mental health professionals ("Functional Overlap Between the Lawyer and Other Professionals," 1962). The psychological equivalent of taking someone's temperature, blood pressure, or X-ray is learning how they are feeling, what they have been doing, and the nature of stressors and crises in their lives. The greater the reluctance to disclose, the greater the likelihood that critical issues and highly relevant history will be unavailable, thereby limiting diagnostic ability and therapeutic opportunities.

Numerous accounts of patients' concerns have been reported to the National Coalition of Mental Health Professionals and Consumers, Inc. (*Educational and Lobbying Kit,* 1993, p. 10):

1. "Henry," a middle-age man with a childhood history of being severely humiliated, requested treatment due to interpersonal problems, including difficulty trusting others. Henry refused to return to treatment when the therapist was required to submit a detailed report about him and his therapy. The therapist finally convinced him to return, and they spent much time discussing what the therapist should write. The report was written and more sessions were authorized, but Henry never returned for treatment. When the therapist called him, Henry said that the experience of having to divulge information to the company was too humiliating for him. (May 1993)

2. A patient was an employee of the managed care insurance company that insured her. The therapist made the required telephone call to register the patient with the managed care company. The reviewer asked the therapist what the patient had said in the first session. The therapist said she would have to get the patient's permission to reveal this information. When the therapist told the patient of this procedure, the patient cried. She feared that people she knew would gain access to this information. The patient said that she would investigate this herself. The therapist was called by the managed care company and told that the patient had given her permission for the therapist to reveal the information, which the patient confirmed. The patient had been told that there would be no coverage without this, and the patient could not afford treatment without coverage. Treatment was authorized for 10 sessions, but the patient dropped out after 2. (May 1996)

3. "Todd," a 46-year-old officer for a pharmaceutical company, became depressed after his 3-year extramarital affair shattered. He demanded of his doctor unequivocal confidentiality—particularly because his affair had been with another man. He was terrified that his employer or his wife would find out if this information were revealed to the insurer. The psychiatrist said that Todd was in "terrible shape" and that he should be hospitalized, but in order to get approval for the hospitalization, the psychiatrist would have to speak with the managed care com-

pany first, and Todd would not allow him to do so. A month later, Todd committed suicide. (May 1996)

MEDICAL RECORDS

Traditionally, health care systems have maintained records for the sole purpose of providing the best possible medical care. The medical record needs to provide those caring for the patient with an accurate assessment of the patient's history, diagnoses, and treatments. Information about changes in the course of an illness and treatments that are successful and those that are not all contribute to important medical decisions about how best to provide quality patient care. Data about the patient and his or her history also are needed to inform those who are unfamiliar with the patient and who must step in during an emergency. Dates of treatment and type of treatment given also are necessary for billing purposes.

The medical record has assumed an additional role. It is still needed in the provision of quality medical care; however, there is pressure for complete access by those not involved in the treatment of the patient but rather whose interest encompasses decisions about cost containment, authorization of treatment, and legitimacy of claims. This places the writer of the record in a conflicted situation. As reported by Dr. Clayton in *The New York Times,*

> Besides being viewed by doctors and hospitals, most patient records are also available to insurers, pharmacists, state health organizations, and researchers. In addition, sometimes employers, life insurance companies, marketing firms, pharmaceutical companies, and others see all or part of these records. (as cited in Leary, 1997, p. A1:1)

The volume of information required by payers to document treatment is growing at an astonishing rate. Insurance and managed care companies are requiring increasing access to patients' records. They view patients' records as a way to evaluate treatment, ensure that treatment occurred, and make decisions about payment. The reality is that the increased pressure on utilization review has resulted in caretakers' spending more time recording data about patient contacts and less time with patients.

The Los Angeles County Outpatient Clinic requires that all clinicians record their patient contact for every 15-minute interval throughout the day. There must also be a note in every patient's chart to corroborate the recorded data. If a reviewer finds a discrepancy, then the billing and a certain percentage of other bills may be disallowed. This development has caused professionals with sophisticated training to spend an enormous amount of time doing paperwork in order to keep the clinic economically alive. In many university settings, clinicians spend as much as 20% of their time coping with these administrative demands, which diminishes their availability for clinical work.

Managed care companies increasingly are requesting access to the total chart and are intruding more and more into the realm of patient care. Lovelace Health Systems, a subsidiary of Cigna in Albuquerque, New Mexico, used chart review to make clinical recommendations (Smith, 1997). They pored through hundreds of medical charts looking for heavy users of medical services. With the concurrence of the patients' primary care physicians, they sent a Zung Depression Scale questionnaire to the patients in question. Only 30% of the patients returned the report. Those who did respond and had high scores on the depression scale were referred to their physicians for treatment of possible depression. Seventy percent of those contacted did not return the questionnaires. Their silence may reflect uneasiness and distrust precipitated by the unsolicited intrusion. The Sara Lee Company asked Lovelace to screen all of the 500 employees at its factory in Las Cruces, New Mexico, for depression to determine whether those who were missing days and performing below par were depressed. This is not the way to provide health care. It is the physician's responsibility to diagnose and treat the patient. For the administrative staff of a managed care company to do so is an absolute invasion of privacy and a violation of its defined role, which does not include clinical responsibility.

The American Psychiatric Association is involved in a long-term, intensive education program to help the public identify symptoms of depression and to encourage people who are exhibiting those symptoms to seek treatment. Education, personal responsibility, and a working therapeutic relationship are some of the keys to seeking and obtaining successful treatment.

Another challenge in today's world is the anticipation that in time all medical records will be computerized. The challenge exists because there is little doubt about the vulnerability of computer records. C.J. Prime of Pahrump, Nevada, bought a used computer; when she booted it up, she found 2,000 patient records from a pharmacy in Tempe, Arizona ("Patient Files Turn Up in Used Computer," 1997). Computers are wonderful machines that allow efficient and easy access to quantities of information. However, abuses abound.

According to a Louis Harris and Equifax poll (1993), 74% of physicians believe that increased computerization in the medical field will weaken confidentiality. According to the same poll, 85% of the general public placed protecting the confidentiality of patients' medical records ahead of providing data on diseases and treatments. Seventy-one percent of Americans believed that "if privacy is to be preserved, the use of computers must be sharply restricted in the future" (Louis Harris & Equifax, 1993).

Mental health professionals are bewildered about what to write in medical charts. There is a recognized need to maintain a careful record to ensure quality care. An accurate record is crucial for proper treatment of a patient in the absence of the regular caregiver. The record also provides a means of quality review. Increasingly, however, records are being written primarily to answer claims review rather than to provide quality care. With this development, there is a parallel decrease in the value of the chart as an important information document. In the service of protecting confidentiality, many clinicians will omit vital information, thus weakening the value of the information.

Clinicians endeavor to limit access to the medical record, arguing that information of a private nature should be segregated and that only basic information be made available to third-party payers. Diagnoses, formulations, and treatment decisions are not made by reviewing charts. They are made by meeting with, interviewing, and examining the patient. The clinician's findings are reported in the chart and reflect the skill, accuracy, and competence of the professional. A report written by this same professional for claims review would be expected to contain the same accuracy but without the inclusion of sensitive and unnecessary intimate personal details. To clear the hurdle of claims review, some professionals who are unclear about the expectations of reviewers offer excessively intimate information. Other clinicians who are aware of the risks of confidentiality breaches attempt to shape the chart entry to meet the most minimal criteria of medical necessity and the *Diagnostic and Statistical Manual of Mental Disorders, Fourth Edition* (DSM-IV; American Psychiatric Association, 1994). Third-party reviewers and clinicians should be able to determine in advance what information is needed for the third party to agree to pay for treatment. Ordinarily, the diagnoses, dates of treatment, types of treatment, goals of treatment, and prognoses are sufficient and can be provided without harmful intrusions.

Records requested for review by accreditation bodies or for investigation of potential fraud can be purged of patient identifiers prior to being made available to reviewers or investigators. There are profound dangers in diverting the medical record from its primary purpose as an instrument useful in the provision of quality health care. As the medical record is forced to act as a resource for claims review and criminal investigation, it will be less and less potent as a useful tool in quality care.

Secretary of the Department of Health and Human Services Donna Shalala's report to the Senate Committee on Labor and Human Resources expressed a deep concern about the protection of medical privacy (*Confidentiality of Individually-Identifiable Health Information,* 1997). She called for harsh penalties for unauthorized disclosures of medical information, stating, "There should be criminal penalties for obtaining health information under false pretenses and for knowingly disclosing or using medical information in violation of the federal privacy laws." But, penalties for abuse will not begin to dispel the concerns of the public.

It is common knowledge in today's world that many knowledgeable computer mavens, including some 10- and 11-year-olds, are able to access sensitive information in computer files. The public will not trust that this can be prevented by the initiation of harsh punishments for illegal entry. People do not feel safe in their homes because their state has enacted the death penalty. They feel safe because of the family that surrounds them, trust in their neighbors, locks on their doors, and police patrolling the neighborhood. Similarly, public trust will not automatically accrue from the initiation of harsh punishments for breaking and entering. Patients' trust accrues from a constant sense of safety within the doctor–patient relationship.

Dangers to patient privacy are being publicized in every newspaper and magazine. In a section entitled "How to Protect Yourself," *Money* magazine recommended, "If possible, don't file for reimbursement from your insurer, and go to a practitioner or druggist who agrees not to report the results to your insurer or employer" (Dowd, 1997)—an interesting and frequently offered recommendation, but not one that most people can afford.

INFORMED CONSENT

The legal doctrine of informed consent is "a hybrid concept which speaks both to physicians' disclosure obligations and patients' willingness to undergo a particular treatment" (Katz, 1994, p. 70). In a 1957 California malpractice case, the court ruled that there is a need to disclose all of the relevant risks and benefits to the patient seeking care from the doctor (*Salgo v. Leland Stanford Junior University Board of Trustees,* 1957). Judge Schroeder's decision in a Kansas case in 1960 attempted to be more specific about the physician's responsibility,

To disclose and explain to the patient, in language as simple as necessary, the nature of the ailment, the nature of the proposed treatment, the probability of success or of alternatives, and perhaps the risks of unfortunate results and unforeseen conditions within the body. (*Natanson v. Kline,* 1960)

There is a basic democratic principle involved in these decisions, which speaks to the issue of autonomy. As Katz wrote, "Underlying the legal doctrine there lurks a broader assumption. . . . That from now on patients and physicians must make decisions jointly, with patients ultimately deciding whether to accede to doctors' recommendations" (1994, p. 80).

This legal doctrine emphasizes the right of the individual to be given the necessary information to make an informed decision. Benefits and side effects of medication, hospitalization, and psychotherapies need to be explained. Individuals assume that, unless otherwise informed, the information that they provide will remain confidential.

Consequently, patients must be told when the opposite is true. For instance, the patient should be informed that the information will not be held in confidence when psychiatric examinations are conducted with the explicit and predetermined purpose of providing information to a court, an insurance company, or a lawyer. Decisions about how much and when to inform are more complex when they involve informing patients about the laws that require reporting of abuse of children or older adults, sexual abuse, and other violence. There are those who at the outset of treatment present patients with a list of the legally required disclosures as well the possible path and exposure that the medical record will encounter. The goal is to achieve a trust in the relationship while dealing openly with the realities of today's world.

Clinicians know that giving an informed consent about the information that must be released to third parties will potentially inhibit patients' communications. Each time they discuss a patient's case with a third-party payer and then must report the interaction to the patient, they see how this interrupts the progress of treatment. Patients become diverted from the work of treatment with questions and concerns about the report and all that it means to them and those who will read it. Some feel as though there is a third party in the room, and it takes time to return to the treatment process with some sense of comfort. Despite these reactions, it is necessary to talk about what has occurred with the third-party payer because to remain silent or secretive damages the patient's trust in the clinician.

Questions are continually raised about whether patients are truly concerned about confidentiality and/or informed consent. Schmid, Applebaum, Roth, and Lidz (1983) found that in a study of 30 psychiatric patients, 80% said that an assurance of confidentiality improved their relationship with the staff, 67% said that they would be upset or angry if verbal information were released without permission, 17% said that they would leave treatment in that event, and 95% were upset at the thought of their charts being released without their consent.

In the climate of pressure for cost containment, informed consent is at great risk. It is viewed by some as an unnecessary impediment, obstructing the efficient management of the business of providing health care. The National Committee on Vital and Health Statistics, which makes recommendations to Shalala, reported, "The extent to which patient authorizations can and should be used as a primary regulatory device for health information disclosure is a major and difficult issue. . . . There is a need . . . to find a procedure that provides effective patient protection in the real world." They concluded that "less insistence on patient authorization could actually result in better patient protections if thoughtful statutory restrictions were placed on specific usages and appropriate accountability imposed" ("Health Privacy and Confidentiality Recommendations of the U.S. Department of Health and Human Services National Committee on Vital and Health Statistics Subcommittee on Privacy and Confidentiality," 1997, p. 10). These recommendations were not made by clinicians. The one clinician on the committee did not vote in support of the recommendations. The others, not working in a clinical setting, were less aware of the therapeutic pitfalls attendant to weakening confidentiality, but the committee's words were then echoed in Shalala's report to Congress (*Confidentiality of Individually-Identifiable Health Information,* 1997). Giving as her rationale that the reality of the present authorization process is that the patient has little actual control of information, she recommended that the traditional control on use and disclosure of information, the patient's written authorization, be replaced by "a system of federal legislative controls on the use of health information collected by health care payers and providers" (p. 6). Again, Shalala was looking to reassure an uneasy public by offering the promise of federal codes and regulations to effect control while undoing the tradition of patient responsibility and autonomy.

Unauthorized release of records for research purposes was also advised by the committee and was included in Shalala's recommendations to the Senate subcommittee. The report read, "We recommend that providers and payers and those receiving information under the provisions of the legislation without patient authorization be permitted to disclose health information without patient authorization for research" (p. 37). Although health research certainly is a priority, the committee indicated that patient consent for release of information for research purposes is impractical and expensive.

What is lost and what is gained by obtaining the patient's permission to use his or her health care information for research purposes? What is lost is convenience. What is gained is cooperation. My personal experience in enlisting patients in a number of clinical studies informs me that a careful and thoughtful discussion of the project, including an explanation that although the project will have no direct value for the patient but might in the future help others, resulted in the majority of patients' eager participation. In one such study, 50 of 51 women who were asked to participate in a study of the psychological sequelae of breast reconstruction following mastectomy for cancer quickly agreed (Goin & Goin, 1981). The data that resulted from this study provided information about psychological distress and patterns of response. Subsequently, physicians were able to help patients by anticipating and reassuring them as problems arose, and other women were helped by the knowledge of what to expect. All of this and other useful interventions were achieved while maintaining the privacy of those who had participated in the study.

A serendipitous finding was some information about the women's reactions to other situations in which information was released without their authorization or informed consent. This was in relation to requests for annual reports about their physical status sent to them from the hospital where they had the original cancer surgery. When requests came from the hospital asking about their health status, the women realized that these were sent because their names had been placed in a cancer data bank for statistical purposes and without their permission. A number of the women told the investigators that they had reacted by tossing the information requests in the trash. They would have the surgery, the chemotherapy, or the radiation, but they rebelled at the intrusion of the statistician who had not asked for their permission.

RELEASE OF MEDICAL RECORDS
TO LAW ENFORCEMENT AGENCIES

Shalala recommended that medical records be made available to intelligence agencies as well as law enforcement officers, "unfettered by new restrictions" (Pear, 1997, p. A24). The report stated,

> We recommend that providers and payers and those receiving informa-
> tion under the provisions of the legislation without patient authoriza-
> tion . . . to disclose health information without patient authorization
> . . . upon request of a law enforcement official who states that
> the health information is needed for a legitimate law enforcement in-
> quiry . . . that the intelligence community and law enforcement agen-
> cies which receive information under this provision not be subject to
> restrictions on its further use or disclosure. (Pear, 1997, p. A24)

These recommendations eliminate requirements for due process, search warrants, and subpoenas. Medical treatment and medical records become an increasing liability and are less and less therapeutic.

THE JUSTICE SYSTEM

Although legislative activity is moving in the direction of stripping away privacy and confidentiality, there have been two Supreme Court decisions that are contrary to Shalala's recommendations. The first case is *Jaffee v. Redmond* (1996). Mary Lou Redmond, an on-duty police officer, responded to a "fight in progress" call for help and was told by two women waving their arms and shouting that there had been a stabbing. Rickie Allen ran out of the apartment brandishing a butcher knife, and when Redmond believed that he was going to stab another man, she shot and killed Allen. After the shooting, she sought counseling from a licensed clinical social worker, Karen Beyer. The administrator of Allen's estate filed an action alleging that Allen's constitutional rights were violated. The court ordered Redmond to give the petitioner notes made by Beyer during the counseling sessions. Both Redmond and Beyer refused to turn over the notes. The jury then awarded the petitioner damages after being instructed that the refusal to turn over the notes was legally unjustified and that the jury could presume that the notes would have been unfavorable to respondents. A Court of Appeals, however, reversed this decision, finding that

> Reason and experience . . . compelled recognition of a psychotherapist–
> patient privilege. Significant private interests support recognition of a
> psychotherapist privilege. Effective psychotherapy depends upon an
> atmosphere of confidence and trust, and therefore the mere possibility
> of disclosure of confidential communications may impede develop-
> ment of the relationship necessary for successful treatment. . . . The
> privilege also serves the public interest, since the mental health of the
> nation's citizenry, no less than its physical health, is a public good of
> transcendent importance.

The appellate decision was upheld by a seven-to-two decision. The Supreme Court commented that the fear of losing information that is important to police investigations was specious because a patient who knew that there was no confidentiality would not disclose such information.

A second case, *Darlene Vasconcellos v. Cybex International* (1997), supported the *Jaffee v. Redmond* decision. Ms. Vasconcellos contended that she was assaulted by a co-worker in the course of her employment with Cybex. She asserted that as a result of this assault, she required immediate medical attention for serious mental and physical health conditions that rendered her unable to perform the functions of her job for a prolonged period of time. The defendants requested the records of Dr. Beth Wadman, who had been Ms. Vasconcellos's treating psychiatrist since shortly after the assault, which gave rise to the lawsuits asserting that Ms. Vasconcellos had waived her privilege by putting her mental condition in issue.

The Court found that

> Ms. Vasconcellos has raised serious concerns that the disclosures will adversely affect her psychiatric treatment by destroying the confidentiality of her relationship with Dr. Wadman. . . . In light of the important public policy behind the existence of the psychotherapist privilege, this is still an important consideration to the Court, *even* if Ms. Vasconcellos has placed her mental state at issue.

The U.S. Federal District judge quashed the subpoena, citing the view of the Supreme Court in *Redmond v. Jaffee* that society must provide a circumstance in which citizens, injured as Officer Redmond was, can find therapeutic help to restore them to health and function, even if mental condition has been brought into issue.

The court also emphasized the importance of not engaging in "fishing expeditions" and commented that there were other means of getting the information that they wanted. Ms. Vasconcellos had volunteered to undergo a psychiatric evaluation as this would not damage her therapeutic relationship.

This is a revolutionary development in the recognition of the right to privacy. Shalala's recommendations are directly antithetical to this increasing jurisprudential recognition at the highest levels of a personal right to confidentiality. The courts appreciate the benefit to the public of maintaining patient privacy. The legislature, caught up with problems of cost containment and law enforcement, fail to realize the loss to the public when mental health professionals are steered away from their role of healing by demands for policing.

CONCLUSION

Given that people have strong privacy concerns that affect their health decisions, informed citizens need to promote legislation that restricts access to medical records. Private citizens, patient coalitions, employers, and employees need to lobby every person in Congress to develop and support legislation that provides appropriately informed consent and privacy protection. If such legislation has not been enacted by August 1999, then the Secretary of the Department of Health and Human Services is required by law to provide such regulations.

If computerized records are to be a future reality, then encryption without trap doors must also be a reality. We must use the best and brightest from the world of technology to turn the advances in the world of technology to our advantage, using them to remove patient identifiers for record reviewers, third-party payers, and researchers.

Punishment for unauthorized disclosures must be enforced, but this is not the ultimate answer. The amount of information made available must be limited.

The criteria for authorizing payment should be known and classified in advance. Mental health professionals can provide the information in a manner separated from the medical chart, thus protecting sensitive and personal information that is not necessary for the authorization process.

Prospective research studies should continue to require patients' informed consent. This is not an impossible task. Informed consent must not be allowed to die. It has had a difficult life, sometimes overworked and at other times forgotten, but its importance remains. Talking with patients helps them to maintain their autonomy. It engenders responsibility and a working relationship, which enhances the process of diagnosis and treatment.

Finally, proposed recommendations to release medical records freely to law enforcement and intelligence agencies must not be allowed to occur. This should not be done until public need has proved to outweigh the needs of personal privacy. Legislators need to match their concerns and efforts with those of the courts and listen carefully to the recent decisions of the justice system. The needs of personal privacy and the impact of continued erosion of these rights far outweigh the perceived public need to know.

REFERENCES

American Psychiatric Association. (1994). *Diagnostic and statistical manual of mental disorders* (4th ed.). Washington, DC: Author.

Cheng, T.L., Savageau, J.A., Sattler, A.L., & DeWitt, T.G. (1993). Confidentiality in health care: A survey of knowledge, perceptions, and attitudes among high school students. *Journal of the American Medical Association, 269,* 1040–1047.

Confidentiality of Individually-Identifiable Health Information. [pursuant to section 264 of the Health Insurance Portability and Accountability Act of 1996] Submitted to: The Committee on Labor and Human Resources and the Committee on Finance of the Senate. The Committee on Commerce and the Committee on Ways and Means of the House of Representatives. (September 11, 1997) (Recommendations of the Secretary of Health and Human Services).

Darlene Vasconcellos v. Cybex International, Inc., ref. 962 F. supp. 701. (U.S. Dist. 1997). Lexis 5087.

Dowd, A.R. (1997, August). Protect your privacy: A *Money* investigation reveals the five biggest threats to your privacy and how you can safeguard yourself against the most serious types of snooping. *Money,* 104–112.

Educational and lobbying kit. (1993). National Coalition of Mental Health Professionals and Consumers, Inc. (Available from the publisher, Post Office Box 438, Commack, NY 11725)

Ford, C., Millstein, S., Halpern-Feisher, B., & Irwin, C. (1997). Influence of physician confidentiality assurances on adolescents' willingness to disclose information and seek future health care. *Journal of the American Medical Association, 278,* 1029–1034.

Functional overlap between the lawyer and other professionals: Its implications for the privileged communications doctrine [Comment]. (1962). *Yale Law Journal, 71,* 1226–1273.

Ginsberg, K.R., Slap, G.B., Cnaan, A., Forke, C.M., Balsley, C.M., & Rouselle, D.M. (1995). Adolescents' perceptions of factors affecting their decisions to seek health care. *Journal of the American Medical Association, 273,* 191–198.

Goin, M.K., & Goin, J.M. (1981). Midlife reactions to mastectomy and subsequent breast reconstruction. *Archives of General Psychiatry, 38,* 225–227.

Health Privacy and Confidentiality Recommendations of the National Committee on Vital and Health Statistics Subcommittee on Privacy and Confidentiality. Approved June 25, 1997.

Jaffee v. Redmond, 64 U.S. L.W. 4490 (Sup. Ct. June 13, 1996).

Katz, J. (1994). Informed consent: Must it remain a fairy tale? *The Journal of Contemporary Health Law and Policy, 10,* 69–91.

Leary, W. (1997, March 6). Panel cites lack of security on medical records. *The New York Times,* p. A1:1.

Lindethal, J.J., & Thomas, C.S. (1982). Psychiatrists, the public and confidentiality. *Journal of Nervous and Mental Disease, 170,* 319–323.

Louis Harris and Associates, Harris. Equifax. (1993). *Health information privacy survey.* New York: Louis Harris and Associates.

McLean, S.A. (1994). Mapping the human genome: Friend or foe? *Social Science and Medicine, 39,* 1221–1227.

Mehlman, M.J., Kodish, E.D., Whitehouse, P., Zinn, A.B., & Sollitto, S. (1996). The need for anonymous genetic counseling and testing. *American Journal of Human Genetics, 58,* 393–397.

Natanson v. Kline, 350, p2d 1093 (Kan. 1960).

On-line medical records raise privacy fears. (1995, March 22). *USA Today.*

Patient files turn up in used computer. (1997, April 4). *The New York Times,* p. 14.

Pear, R. (1997, September 12). Limited access to medical records is urged. *The New York Times,* p. A24.

Rothstein, M.A. (1995). Genetic testing: Employability, insurability and health reform. *Monographs of the National Cancer Institute, 17,* 87–90.

Report to Congress. *Testimony before the senate committee on labor and human resources,* 105th Cong., 1st Sess. (1997, September 11) (testimony of D.E. Shalala).

Salgo v. Leland Stanford Jr. University Board of Trustees, 387 P.2d (Cal. Dist. Ct. App. 1957)

Schmid, D., Applebaum, P.S., Roth, L.H., & Lidz, C. (1983). Confidentiality in psychiatry: A study of the patient's view. *Hospital and Community Psychiatry, 34,* 353–355.

Shore, D., Berg, K., Wynne, D., & Folstein, M.F. (1993, May 1). Legal and ethical issues in psychiatric genetic research. *American Journal of Medical Genetics, 48*(1), 17–21.

Smith, L. (1997, May 12). It's not creepy—it's a wonder drug: Can Prozac cut health costs? *Fortune,* 28.

What to watch for in health care reform. (1994, June). *Consumer Reports,* 396–398.

Woodard, B. (1995). Sounding board: The computer-based patient record and confidentiality. *New England Journal of Medicine, 333,* 4119–4122.

6

Legal and Ethical Issues in Protecting the Privacy of Behavioral Health Care Information

John Petrila

Confidentiality of health care information is a core ethical principle. The Hippocratic Oath states that "whatever in connection with my professional practice, or not in connection with it, I see or hear in the life of men, which ought not to be spoken of abroad, I will not divulge, as reckoning that all such should be kept secret." Contemporary ethical canons of the various health care professions articulate the same principle. For example, the Code of Medical Ethics of the American Medical Association says that "a physician . . . shall safeguard a patient's confidences within the restraints of the law" (American Medical Association, Council on Ethical and Judicial Affairs, 1997). The confidentiality of health care information is also a core legal principle. All states and the federal government have statutes protecting confidentiality. Both state and federal courts have endorsed its importance.

Certain types of health care information are considered sufficiently sensitive to warrant special protection. For example, nearly all states have separate statutes that make confidential mental health and substance abuse information. Stringent federal protections govern the confidentiality of information gained in providing substance abuse treatment. Similarly, all states have separate statutes providing for the confidentiality of information regarding individuals with HIV or AIDS.

Despite its importance as an ethical and legal principle, the confidentiality of health care information is not an absolute value. There are circumstances in which both law and ethics permit or require confidentiality to be breached. For example, the ethical principles of the American Psychological Association (1992) permit the disclosure of otherwise confidential information "where permitted by law for a valid purpose, such as . . . to protect the patient or client from harm." An example of a mandated breach of confidentiality is the obligation, imposed by all states, to report suspected child abuse.

Dramatic changes in the financing and delivery of health care and behavioral health care services, combined with advances in the technology for storing and transmitting information, have led to new concerns regarding the confidentiality of health care information. Most Americans consider their health status and experience as patients to be deeply personal. At the same time, many Americans are increasingly concerned that information regarding their health status is subject to scrutiny and use by individuals and organizations far removed from the treatment process. In fact, a Harris poll conducted at the request of Equifax, an Atlanta-based company that furnishes consumer information for commercial transactions, found that approximately one quarter of Americans believed that health care information had been improperly disclosed during claims transactions and that nearly two thirds were concerned that organizations not involved in their health care were obtaining access to health care information (Peck, 1994).

In response, a consensus has begun to form that the current statutory, regulatory, and judicial framework protecting confidentiality is inadequate. A number of bills have been introduced in Congress to create a national confidentiality standard. In addition, Congress, as part of the Health Insurance Portability and Accountability Act (HIPAA) of 1996 (PL 104-191), directed the Secretary of the Department of Health and Human Services (DHHS) to make recommendations in 1997 regarding the privacy of health care information. In the same statute, Congress determined that if it did not enact legislation by August 1999 (36 months from the effective date of HIPAA), then the Secretary of the DHHS would promulgate federal regulations. The likely development of federal standards has sharpened the debate regarding confidentiality.

This chapter has four sections. The first section discusses the values underlying the confidentiality of mental health and substance abuse information. The second section summarizes pertinent statutory provisions and judicial rulings that form the legal basis for confidentiality of behavioral health care information as well as exceptions to that principle. The third section describes the debate regarding the need for a national standard and a general description of the core issues in that debate. The final section delineates the policy choices that the mental health and substance abuse communities face in considering ways to strengthen the protection of behavioral and general health care information.

A note on terminology as used in this chapter may be helpful. The term *confidentiality* rather than *privacy* is used most frequently because most state laws choose the former rather than the latter term, though *privacy* increasingly is becoming the term of art. Second, *health care information* is used more frequently than *the health care record* because it has become increasingly obvious that information regarding individual health status is often created and held outside the clinical relationship. Although most confidentiality laws are written to protect what occurs within the health care relationship, most reform proposals seek to ensure confidentiality and to minimize invasions of privacy when the information generated is held by secondary and tertiary users. Finally, the term *behavioral health care* is used occasionally as a proxy for mental health, substance abuse, and alcohol abuse treatment combined. When *substance abuse* is used, it includes alcohol abuse as well.

VALUES UNDERLYING CONFIDENTIALITY

The legal protection of confidentiality rests on four values: stigma, trust, privacy, and autonomy.

Stigma

Individuals with mental illness and substance abuse disorders historically have encountered discrimination. Until the mental health law revolution of the late 1960s and 1970s, that discrimination was often legally enforced. In many states, individuals hospitalized for mental health treatment automatically became legally incompetent, losing rights to vote, to contract, to execute a will, and to make treatment decisions. Legal rules now exist to protect the rights of people with mental disabilities—examples include the Americans with Disabilities Act (ADA) of 1990 (PL 101-336) and the Fair Housing Amendments Act of 1988 (PL 100-430), as well as state and federal legislation designed to achieve parity in insurance coverage of mental and physical health. However, stigma and discrimination are still issues for people seeking treatment for mental disabilities. The law assumes that the risk of stigma can be partially ameliorated if an individual has some assurance that disclosures made during treatment will remain private.

Trust

Many psychotherapists recognize that mental health treatment, particularly verbal therapies, can proceed only when there is trust between the therapist and the client. The ability to foster trust depends, in turn, on protecting from the scrutiny of others what occurs in the clinical relationship. Without such protection, it is argued, individuals will not reveal themselves during treatment. In 1996, the U.S. Supreme Court joined the courts and legislatures that have endorsed this belief. Holding that there is a federal psychotherapist privilege, the Supreme Court's majority observed that

> Effective psychotherapy . . . depends upon an atmosphere of confidence and trust in which the patient is willing to make a frank and complete disclosure of facts, emotions, memories, and fears . . . the mere possibility of disclosure may impede development of the confidential relationship necessary for successful treatment. (*Jaffee v. Redmond,* 1996)

Privacy

Since the 1960s, the courts have concluded that individuals have significant privacy rights regarding health care and other personal decisions. Although these decisions have most notably involved procreation, as well as death and dying, the importance of privacy in seeking other types of treatment, including mental health and substance abuse treatment, has been acknowledged as well. Privacy may be particularly important in the context of mental health treatment. This is because of the stigma often associated with mental illness and because in treatment the individual may literally reveal secrets about him- or herself.

Autonomy

The value of privacy is closely related to the value of autonomy in health care decision making. Competent individuals have a right to self-determination in deciding to seek or forego health care, including mental health and substance abuse treatment. Debates regarding confidentiality have suggested that an important part of exercising autonomy in health care decision making is knowing the extent of third-party access to health care information. That is, a person's concerns regarding potential intrusions into privacy might cause that individual to decide not to seek health care or at least to pay for it privately (Patterson, 1989).

Integrity of the Values Underlying Confidentiality

Although each of the values underlying confidentiality has received strong legal endorsement, the confidentiality of health care information is not absolute, and intrusions into privacy may be growing. The Institute of Medicine (Donaldson & Lohr, 1994) identified more than 60 different uses of health care information. At the same time, not all parties who have access to health care information have equal footing. Alan Westin, a noted privacy expert, categorizes those with access to personal health care information into three "zones." Zone 1 users are involved in direct patient care. Zone 2 users are engaged in support and administrative activities—for example, payers, administrators, and quality-of-care reviewers. Zone 3 users include recipients of public health reporting, social welfare agencies, researchers, and direct marketing firms (Schwartz, 1995). Some of these users, such as those providing care, public health officials, and researchers, traditionally have had access. Others, such as utilization review managers and direct marketing firms, are comparatively new players on the health care field. Much of the debate today focuses on which types of users should have which types of access to health care information. Another way to frame the same question is, "When should private or public interests in obtaining access outweigh individual privacy interests?"

There have also been dramatic advances in the technology of record keeping. Gostin (1996) identified three innovations that have accelerated the pace of automation. The first is the development of longitudinal health records, which capture a person's health care history from prenatal care to death. It is worth noting that with the rapid advances in the field of genetics, these longitudinal records will soon be intergenerational. The second is that most health care reform proposals would assign an individual health care identifier to each American to facilitate the exchange and transmission of health care information. The debate is not over whether such identifiers should be assigned but whether identifiers such as social security numbers or identifiers based on DNA samples (Dahm, 1997) should be used for this purpose. Finally, advanced technology makes it feasible to store and rapidly transmit large quantities of data across state and national boundaries. In fact, it is often argued that the cost-efficient management of health care requires the use of such technology. This technology and the manner in which claims data are bundled and transmitted rapidly across state borders have added weight to the argument that discrete state laws are no longer adequate to regulate the confidentiality of health care information.

Although these changes do not necessarily mean that individual privacy will be invaded, the use of individual health care information for purposes that may compromise individual privacy interests appears to be growing and has led to increased public apprehension about how well health care information is protected (Schwartz, 1995). A particular concern has been the emergence of the collection and selling of private health care information for business purposes, projected to grow into an $8.8 billion industry (*Confidentiality of Medical Information,* 1997).

LEGAL RULES GOVERNING CONFIDENTIALITY OF MENTAL HEALTH AND SUBSTANCE ABUSE INFORMATION

The laws governing the confidentiality of mental health and substance abuse treatment information are an uneasy mixture of state and federal statutory, regulatory, and judicial law. A key distinction between the regulation of the confidentiality of mental health information and the regulation of substance abuse information is that the former is governed almost exclusively by state law, whereas the latter is governed by very explicit federal standards.

State Mental Health Confidentiality Laws

Each state has a statute addressing the confidentiality of general health care information. Most states also have a separate statute defining the confidentiality of mental health and substance abuse records and information. There appear to be at least two reasons for this. First, each state has for its mental health system a statutory base that is distinct from the statutory base for public health issues, and so confidentiality, as an important mental health issue, is treated within the state's mental health law. Second, discrete protections for mental health and substance abuse treatment records may reflect a judgment that such information requires more protection than general health care information. An important issue in debates regarding confidentiality is whether these distinctions should be maintained, a topic discussed in more detail below.

The features of a typical state mental health confidentiality statute are discussed in the sections that follow. (*Note:* Many states also include protections for information generated during substance abuse treatment; however, because federal law mandates that state law be at least as strong as the federal alcohol and substance abuse confidentiality provisions, the following discussion of state law focuses on mental health issues.)

Definition of the Principle of Confidentiality A state mental health confidentiality statute usually begins with the principle that records and other information gathered in treatment are confidential and are not to be disclosed absent a legislatively or judicially created exception. For example, Alaska's mental health law provides that "information and records obtained in the course of a screening investigation, evaluation, examination, or treatment are confidential and are not public records," with exceptions noted in the statute (Alaska Stat. § 47.30.845 [1996]). The Delaware law provides that "no information reported to the [mental health] Department and no clinical records maintained with respect to patients shall be public records . . . [and] shall not be released" except pursuant to exceptions set forth in the statute (16 Del. Laws 5161[13] [1995]). Note that these definitions focus on material obtained during clinical interactions; state laws may but often do not apply to health care information generated or obtained by other entities—for example, payers and employers. This is a deficiency that most reform proposals attempt to remedy.

Exceptions to Confidentiality After creating a general principle of confidentiality, all state laws then create a list of exceptions. The most common are discussed next. There are significant differences among the states in the types and definitions of exceptions to confidentiality.

Patient Consent A competent client may consent to the disclosure of health care information in all states. For example, a client may wish to have information released to another treatment provider; in such a situation, the current provider will have the client sign a form consenting to this disclosure. Although all state laws discuss client consent as an exception to confidentiality, many state statutes provide little guidance on what constitutes an adequate consent. For example, Tennessee law provides simply that "any of the following may consent: (a) the individual identified who is sixteen (16) years of age or over; (b) the legal guardian. . .; (c) the parent, guardian, or custodian of a minor; (d) the executor, administrator, or personal representative" (Tenn. Code Ann. § 33-3-104[10] [1998]). The Wisconsin statute, in contrast, defines in some detail the elements of consent to disclosure:

> An informed consent for disclosure . . . must be in writing and must contain the following: the name of the individual, agency, or organization to which the disclosure is to be made; the name of the individual whose treatment record is being disclosed; the purpose or need of the disclosure; the specific type of information to be disclosed; the time period during which the consent is effective; the date on which the consent is signed; and the signature of the individual or person legally authorized to give consent for the individual. (Wis. Stat. Ann. § 51.30[2] [West 1997])

The federal substance abuse regulations and most reform proposals provide more detailed information regarding a legally sufficient consent than is found in most state mental health laws.

Other Treatment Providers   An individual who is being treated for mental illness often will be treated by more than one provider. Most practitioners assume that the individual must consent before information is made available to another provider. However, state laws are inconsistent on the question of whether consent must be obtained prior to disclosure to another provider. Some states permit disclosure to other treatment providers without client consent. Others require client consent before disclosure, and still others do not address the topic. Those states permitting disclosure without consent may limit the types of providers that can receive information. For example, New York provides for disclosure between providers without patient consent if the providers are part of an "approved local or unified services plan . . . or pursuant to agreement with the [mental health] department" (N.Y. Mental Hyg. Law § 33.13[d] [McKinney 1996]).

Wisconsin permits disclosure within the department responsible for behavioral health treatment as necessary to coordinate treatment for individuals committed to or under the supervision of the department; to facilities receiving individuals who are involuntarily committed, with limitations on the types of information conveyed; to correctional facilities or probation and parole officers in certain circumstances; and to county departments responsible for coordinating care (Wis. Stat. Ann. § 51.30 [4][b] 5, 7, 9, 10, 15 [West 1997]). Pennsylvania law is more general:

> Whenever a person who has previously received services or benefits at a facility is later given services or benefits at another facility, the first facility shall, upon request from the subsequent facility, furnish a copy of all pertinent records pertaining to such person. (50 Pa. Code § 4602[c] [1998])

The emergence of managed care has resulted in the creation of provider networks. These networks, often linked by contract, may result in the treatment of an individual by a variety of providers within a single course of treatment. The question of whether consent should be required for disclosures of information within the network is one on which there are a variety of opinions. Some believe that consent should be required as part of the exercise of patient autonomy; others believe that a network of providers should be treated as a single provider for purposes of disclosure during a single course of treatment. State laws typically do not address the issue, probably because state confidentiality laws were written before the emergence of managed care.

Reimbursement   Payers of health care services want to know that the services for which they are paying were appropriate clinically. Insurance contracts and managed care contracts often state that services will be paid for only if they are "medically necessary." In making this determination, payers traditionally have required some information from the clinician justifying the particular service or intervention in question. However, as managed care has emerged, payers have demanded significantly more information from health care professionals, raising questions about the intrusion into patient confidentiality that such requests represent.

As noted previously, most state laws were written before the emergence of managed care and so rarely limit the amount of information that payers can request in making reimbursement decisions. In fact, many states allow a provider to make any disclosure necessary to obtain reimbursement without the consent of the client. For example, the Texas mental health code permits disclosure of confidential information by mental health professionals "to individuals, corporations, or governmental agencies involved in paying or collecting fees for mental or emotional health services provided by a professional" (Tex. Health & Safety Code Ann. § 611.004[6] [West Supp. 1998]). Colorado permits disclosure "to the extent necessary to make claims on behalf of a recipient of aid, insurance, or medical assistance to which he may be entitled" (Colo. Rev. Stat. Ann. § 27-10-120[1][c] [West 1990]). Illinois law exempts insurance companies and nonprofit health care service plan corporations from the general consent requirements of the Illinois mental health law and permits such companies to obtain "general consents for the release to them or their designated representatives of any and all confidential information" (Ill. Ann. Stat. 740 110/5[f] [Smith-Hurd 1998]).

As the discussion of reform proposals next suggests, the question of what kinds of restrictions, if any, should exist regarding the transmission of information to payers is a closely debated issue.

Disclosures to Families   Families often play an important caregiving role for people with mental illness. Often, an individual lives with his or her family while receiving treatment. A common complaint of families is that they receive too little information from mental health professionals regarding the condition and treatment of the individual residing with them (Petrila, 1992). Their view is that information necessary for them to play a caregiver role should be made available even if the individual does not consent. Conversely, some spokespersons for individuals with mental illness believe that consent should be a necessary prerequisite before information is given to families.

A handful of states have amended their mental health confidentiality laws to permit some information to be made available to family members who are acting in the role of caregiver. For example, New Hampshire law provides that a community mental health center or state facility

> May disclose information regarding diagnosis, admission to or discharge from a treatment facility, functional assessment, the name of the medicine prescribed, the side effects of any medication prescribed, behavioral or physical manifestations which would result from failure of the client to take such prescribed medication, treatment plans and goals and behavioral management strategies to a family member or other person, if such family member or person lives with the client or provides direct care to the client. (N.H. Rev. Stat. Ann. § 135-C:19-aI [1996])

The client is to be asked for written consent, but if consent is not given, disclosure may proceed and the client is to be informed of the reason for disclosure, the information released, and the identity of the recipient. Maine has a similar provision that permits disclosure

> To a family member or other person if the family member or other person lives with or provides direct care to the client, if without the disclosure there would be significant deterioration in the client's daily functioning and if the disclosure is in the best interest of the client. (Me. Rev. Stat. Ann. tit. 34-B § 1207.5 [West Supp. 1998])

The statute provides that the family must request information in writing. The client may deny the request, and the family may appeal the denial to the mental health department. Disclosures are limited to information regarding diagnosis, admission to or discharge from a treatment facility, the name and side effects of prescribed medication, the likely consequences if medication is not taken, and treatment plan goals and behavioral management strategies.

Quality Control/Program Evaluation/Oversight   All states reserve the authority to review patient records without consent to monitor treatment programs, quality issues, and compliance with regulatory requirements. For example, Rhode Island provides for the release of information "for program evaluation and/or research, provided that the director adopts rules for the conduct of the evaluations and/or research" (R.I. Gen. Laws § 40.1-5-26[6] [1997]). Washington's code permits disclosure "to the department of health for the purposes of determining compliance with state or federal licensure, certification, or registration rules or laws" (Wash. Rev. Code § 71.05.390[14] [1998]). State statutes also generally stipulate that individuals conducting program evaluations or quality assurance reviews must promise in writing not to redisclose patient-identifying information.

Research   Some types of research—for example, epidemiological studies or studies of the utilization of health care services—require access to large numbers of health care records. State laws generally do not require individual consent before this type of research may proceed if there are adequate assurances that the research project will not use information in a way that enables an individual to be identified. The specificity of the statutory provisions addressing access for research varies. For example, North Dakota law permits disclosure to "persons doing research or maintaining health statistics if the anonymity of the patient is assured and the facility recognizes the project as a bona fide research or statistical undertaking" (N.D. Cent. Code § 25-03.1-44[5] [1997]). Wyoming law, in contrast, is more detailed, permitting disclosure for research if an institutional review board (IRB) has made several findings, including that the research is sufficiently important to outweigh the intrusion into privacy, is impracticable without disclosure of individually identifiable information, has adequate safeguards to prevent redisclosure and the identification of any subject, and provides for the destruction of identifying information as soon as possible unless the IRB finds that retention is necessary to the project (Wyo. Stat. § 35-2-609[vii] [1997]). Wyoming law is closer to the provisions of most of the federal proposals that have been introduced in recent years.

Public Health Reporting   All states also provide for certain types of information to be made available to public health officials without consent. Examples include the HIV status of an individual (though the states differ on how much and what types of information are to be reported; see Barron, Goldstein, & Wishnev, 1995; State Statutes, 1996) and the prescription of certain types of medications. In the former example, the information is made available to make possible the tracking of an epidemic, a traditional public health function; in the latter, the information is made available to monitor the prescription of medications that have been abused in the past. Courts consistently have upheld public health reporting requirements against challenges that such reporting invades personal privacy, as long as the public agency charged with receiving the information makes reasonable assurances that the information will be secure from unauthorized scrutiny (see, e.g., the discussion of the Supreme Court's decision in *Whalen v. Roe* (1977) in the section "Relevant Supreme Court Cases").

Disclosures to Protect Third Parties   An individual who is in treatment for mental illness may tell his or her therapist that he or she intends to harm another person. The threat may be explicit (e.g., "I'm going to kill my wife if she ever tells me I can't go out with my friends again"). It may be less direct (e.g., "There are times when I just want to punch my boss in the face"; "When I'm riding a crowded subway train, I wish I carried a gun so I could keep people from touching me"). The legal and ethical question in such circumstances is whether the therapist has an obligation to "do something" to prevent the threat from being carried out.

The California Supreme Court, in *Tarasoff v. Regents of University of California* (1976), ruled that a mental health professional who reasonably concludes that his or her client may cause harm to an identified third party must take steps to protect that third party. Since this decision, many states have addressed the obligations of mental health professionals to third parties who might be endangered by a client. However, the approaches vary. The primary difference is how much discretion clinicians enjoy in determining whether to take steps to protect a third party. For example, some states have enacted legislation that permits—but does not require—the therapist to take steps to protect a third party. In those states, the professional judgment of the therapist governs, and a decision to act to protect a third party will not lead to a lawsuit for breach of confidentiality. Conversely, a decision not to take steps to protect a third party is also unlikely to lead to successful litigation, absent a gross departure from professional standards in reaching the underlying clinical judgment, because the point of this type of statute is to make the decision to breach confidentiality a matter of professional judgment, not mandatory duty. For example, in Florida, a mental health professional may but is not required to breach confidentiality if a client has made an actual threat to physically harm an identifiable victim and it is the clinician's professional judgment that the client is capable of committing the act and is more likely than not to do so (Fla. Stat. Ann. Ch. 15, 455.2415 [West 1998]).

In other states, the obligation to take steps to protect the third party provides the clinician with considerably less discretion. For example, the Ohio Supreme Court found that therapists are obligated to take steps to protect the public from clients who they believe are dangerous (*Morgan v. Fairfield Family Counseling Center,* 1997), subordinating the value of protecting confidentiality to the value of protecting an endangered third party. The Ohio court went even further than most of the courts that have created a mandatory duty: Most states in this category limit the duty to identified or identifiable third parties; however, the Ohio Supreme Court appears to have extended the duty to the public at large, a ruling with quite significant ramifications for clinicians in that state. Still other states have rejected the rule that therapists in outpatient settings have any obligation to third parties, principally on the ground that therapists who perform outpatient treatment have little physical control over clients. In any state, therapists must refer to the state confidentiality law as well as to judicial decisions applying the law to determine whether breaches to protect third parties are permitted or required. It should be noted that in all states a mental health facility has an obligation not to act negligently in discharging an individual into the community. Even in states that do not require mental health professionals in an outpatient setting to protect or warn third parties, an inpatient facility may be liable for the negligent discharge of a patient. The difference in the view of the courts that have considered this question is that inpatient facilities have physical control over individuals who are hospitalized there.

The question of whether confidentiality may be breached to prevent the suicide of a client is a discrete question. In most jurisdictions, it has been assumed that such a breach is warranted. A case decided by the Supreme Court of Hawaii reached a different conclusion. The court held that therapists in Hawaii have no obligation to prevent the suicide of a patient who is not within their custody and that imposing such a duty would be objectionable in part because Hawaii law created a preference for the confidentiality of communications between therapists and clients (*Lee v. Corregedore,* 1996).

Another situation in which state laws are explicit regarding disclosure to protect third parties is when an individual is HIV positive and a known sexual partner is to be notified. These laws usually are very specific in structuring disclosure—in general, the treating physician is first to attempt to persuade the patient to disclose his or her status voluntarily; failing that, states provide for disclosure either through the treating physician or through the local public health official.

Disclosures to Law Enforcement Agencies   The question of how much information can be revealed to law enforcement officials is a complex one. As the discussion of the following proposed national legislation suggests, some advocate broad access by law enforcement to address questions such as Medicare fraud. Others believe that access needs to be more limited, on the basis that medical records can become a source for "fishing expeditions" by law enforcement agencies.

There is little uniformity among the states in addressing access to behavioral health information. Some states explicitly permit certain types of disclosures to law enforcement agencies—for example, to assist in locating a missing person. State laws are less clear regarding the appropriate course of conduct when the client may have been involved in a crime. When a client indicates that he or she intends to commit a crime in the future, it is generally assumed that a mental health professional may breach confidentiality (i.e., notify law enforcement) to attempt to prevent the crime from being committed. Massachusetts law is one of the few to address explicitly both past and future criminal conduct, providing that confidentiality of mental health communications is waived "when the communication reveals the contemplation or commission of a crime or a harmful act" (Mass. Ann. Laws, Ch. 112, § 172 [Lawyers Cooperative Publishing, 1985]).

In other situations, disclosure of clinical information is required. The most notable example is when child abuse (and in many states, elder abuse) is suspected. In all states, the mental health professional has an obligation to breach confidentiality and report his or her suspicions to the relevant authorities.

Disclosures to Counsel   As a general rule, state laws permit disclosure of confidential information to attorneys representing clients. This is to permit the attorney to prepare his or her client's case. If the attorney did not have access to information regarding mental status or, when pertinent, treatment history, then he or she might have difficulty in litigating legal issues that turned on such information. For example, if competency to execute a will is at issue, then the mental state of the author of the will at the time that it was written is a core concern in determining whether the person had the necessary competence to write the will.

Disclosures in Court Proceedings and the Question of Privilege   In nearly all states, the question of what type of mental health (and general health) information may be disclosed in court-related proceedings is an amalgam of statutory and judicial law. If the individual has put his or her mental state at issue, then confidentiality may be breached without the individual's consent. For example, if an individual pleads the insanity defense in a criminal case, then the prosecution will be able to discover treatment-related information to contest the claim. The reason for this rule is fairness: If an individual chooses to claim that his or her mental condition has some legal significance, either in a criminal or a civil setting, then the other party is given access to material about the individual's mental state insofar as it is relevant to the legal proceeding. It is also generally assumed that otherwise confidential information regarding a person's mental state and psychiatric history is available in an involuntary civil commitment proceeding.

In other contexts, an individual's mental health record may be subpoenaed, either by an opposing attorney or by the court. For example, in a child custody dispute, one spouse may claim that the fact that his or her spouse has been treated for mental illness makes that spouse an unfit parent. In attempting to prove this claim, the spouse who is making the allegation may attempt to subpoena the person's mental health records to introduce them in the custody dispute. The judge then will have to rule whether such information is of value in the particular custody dispute at issue.

Most states also distinguish between a subpoena that is issued by an attorney and one that is issued by the court. Attorneys routinely subpoena (i.e., send a document demanding) information that they believe might be useful in a legal proceeding. When mental health information is sought through an attorney's subpoena, most states provide that the party receiving the subpoena does not have to honor it. This is because mental health information is considered sufficiently sensitive that state law requires a neutral party—that is, the court—to consider whether the demands of justice in the particular case outweigh the privacy interests of the individual in maintaining the confidentiality of the information. Generally, court orders cannot be ignored. However, even in the face of a court order, the client, the client's attorney, or the client's therapist can claim that the material sought is privileged. If material is privileged, then it cannot be disclosed in court. The underlying reason for such a privilege is that preservation of confidentiality is more important than the evidentiary value of the disputed material. The existence and scope of a privilege in a state is usually a matter of legislative law, whereas the courts determine application of the privilege. An example of a judicially created privilege is the psychotherapist–patient privilege in federal court, an issue discussed in the summary of the decision in *Jaffee v. Redmond* (1996) in the section "Relevant Supreme Court Cases."

Disclosures to the Client   Many states' laws permit a client access to his or her record. Often, the clinician is permitted to redact certain material—for example, material provided in confidence by a third party—prior to making access available. Delaware's statute is typical. A patient's record and information regarding care may be released

To patients or, if the patient is a minor, to a parent or legal guardian, except that access to specific records may be refused when a clinical determination is made and documented in the patient's individualized treatment plan that such access would be seriously detrimental to the patient's health or treatment progress. In the latter case, such material

> may be made available to a licensed mental health professional se-
> lected by the patient, and that professional may, in the exercise of pro-
> fessional judgment, provide the patient with access to any or all parts
> of the denied material or otherwise disclose the information contained
> therein. (16 Del. Laws 5161[13])

Statutes that permit the clinician to redact material or deny access have been criticized by some as paternalistic (Feenan, 1996). The principle of patient access for the purpose of review and correction of errors is part of all proposals to reform confidentiality law.

As this brief review suggests, state laws governing the confidentiality of mental health information differ significantly. In contrast, a single federal standard governs access to substance and alcohol abuse treatment information.

Federal Mental Health Confidentiality Law

Federal Alcohol and Substance Abuse Law   Congress has established special rules for the confidentiality of any information that would identify an individual as receiving substance or alcohol abuse treatment in the Public Health Services Act (PL 102-321; 42 C.F.R. 2.1 *et seq*). These rules assume that strict confidentiality is required to create an incentive for people to seek treatment for substance abuse disorders. In addition, because many behaviors associated with substance abuse are crimes, Congress determined that people would be reluctant to seek treatment if the communications made in the course of treatment could be used as the basis for criminal prosecution.

The statute and implementing regulations apply to a "federally assisted" alcohol or drug abuse program.[1] The statute strictly regulates the disclosure of "patient identifying information," defined as

> The name, address, social security number, fingerprints, photograph, or
> similar information by which the identity of a patient can be deter-
> mined with reasonable accuracy and speed either directly or by refer-
> ence to other publicly available information. The term does not include

---

[1]A program is "federally assisted" if it has a contract with the U.S. government; is licensed or otherwise authorized by an agency of the U.S. government, including certification as a Medicare provider, authorized to conduct methadone maintenance, or registered to dispense a substance under the Controlled Substances Act of 1970 (PL 91-513) to the extent that the substance is used in treating alcohol or substance abuse; is supported by any federal funding, which includes treating recipients of federal assistance or being conducted by state or local government that receives federal funds that could be spent for the alcohol or drug abuse program; or is tax exempt under federal law (42 C.F.R. § 2.12).

a number assigned to a patient by a program, if that number does not consist of or contain numbers (e.g., a social security or driver's license number) which could be used to identify a patient with reasonable accuracy and speed from sources external to the program. (§ 2.11[b])

Although disclosure of otherwise confidential information is permitted, the rules for disclosure are much more explicit and specific than most state mental health confidentiality statutes. As is the case with most state mental health laws, a client may consent to disclosure of information; unlike most state mental health laws, the federal rules dictate in detail what constitutes a valid consent form (§ 2.31[a]).

The statute and regulations permit other types of disclosures as well but strictly define in each case the conditions that must be met before disclosure can occur. Provided that statutory and regulatory conditions are met, disclosures may be made without client consent in the following situations:

- Within the treatment program, when necessary to provide services
- To other providers, pursuant to a "qualified service agreement"
- To report a crime on the program's premises or against treatment personnel
- In medical emergencies
- To report child abuse
- For research and program audits
- In response to court orders
- In criminal investigations when there is an "extremely serious crime" and disclosure is in the public interest

Disclosures to families are not permitted, and the regulations do not explicitly permit disclosure to payers of treatment services.

The conditions for each of these exceptions are not included here but may be found in the implementing regulations, as well as in the Technical Assistance Publications Series (U.S. Department of Health and Human Services, Center for Substance Abuse Treatment, 1994).

As noted, this statutory and regulatory scheme is more detailed than most state mental health statutes. State laws on the confidentiality of alcohol and substance abuse information and records must minimally comply with these federal rules. However, state laws governing the release of mental health records are not bound by these requirements. As this review suggests, the differences between state mental health laws, combined with differences between those laws and federal substance abuse laws, make it difficult at a conceptual level to describe the current standard for the protection of behavioral health care information. It is most accurate to say that beyond the generally accepted principle that behavioral health information should presumptively be confidential, there is no widely agreed-on set of principles that applies across states.

Other Federal Statutes Applicable to Medical Records   At least three other federal statutes apply to medical records, in addition to the HIPAA (which is discussed in more detail in the section "Federal Initiatives"). The first is the Privacy Act of 1974 (PL 93-579). It applies to federally operated hospitals and to research or health care institutions operated pursuant to federal contracts. The Privacy Act prohibits disclosure of information to any person or agency without the individual's prior written consent and permits the individual to review, copy, and correct records. Most commentators believe that this statute has limited utility in ensuring the confidentiality of health care records for two reasons. First, the Privacy Act does not apply to the vast majority of entities collecting health information outside the federal government (Gostin, 1996). Second, the Privacy Act permits disclosure of personally identifiable information to another agency if the information is deemed necessary for the "routine use" of the receiving agency. This is a very broad exception, which invites routine disclosure of information. (Other exceptions to the Privacy Act include disclosure to agency employees who need the record for performing their duties; to the Bureau of the Census; for statistical or research purposes if the record is unidentifiable; to the National Archives; to another agency for civil or criminal law enforcement; to a person showing "compelling circumstances" affecting health or safety; to Congress; to the Comptroller General pursuant to a court order; and to a consumer reporting agency (§ a[b][1]-[12]).)

A second statute of limited applicability is the Freedom of Information Act (FOIA) of 1964 (PL 89-554). The FOIA exempts from discovery "privileged or confidential data" (exemption 4) and "personnel and medical files" if the disclosure would invade personal privacy (exemption 6). In both situations, the agency holding the data may but is not required to claim an exemption from discovery.

Finally, the ADA has some relevance. The ADA requires employers to keep medical information on separate forms and in separate medical files and to treat such information as "a confidential medical record" (§ 12112[c][3] and [4]). However, it is not clear that the ADA has resulted in the elimination of the use of health care information in personnel files to make employment decisions, and it therefore provides uncertain protection of the privacy of health care information.

Medicare rules also require providers to keep patient records confidential. These provisions are found in the federal regulations and apply to different categories of providers—for example, hospitals (§ 482.24[b][3]), home health agencies (§ 484.48[b]), long-term care facilities (§ 483.420[a][7]), outpatient rehabilitation facilities (§ 485.56[c][5]), and rural primary care hospitals (§ 485.638[b]).

Relevant Supreme Court Cases   At least two Supreme Court cases are worth noting. In *Whalen v. Roe* (1977), the Supreme Court upheld the legality of a New York statute that required physicians to provide the state with information regarding prescriptions for specific types of drugs with a high potential for abuse. These data were then stored in a computer. The law was challenged on the grounds that it violated individual privacy. While noting "the threat to privacy implicit in the accumulation of vast amounts of personal information in computerized data banks or other massive government files," the Supreme Court also ruled that New York had created procedures and standards adequate to protect the privacy of the files. Although this decision acknowledges the significance of an individual's interest in the privacy of medical information and the importance of privacy as a cornerstone of autonomous health care decision making, it also gives broad latitude, particularly to public health officials, in collecting information deemed necessary to protect the public health.

In another case, the Supreme Court strongly endorsed the need for privacy in the therapeutic relationship and created a psychotherapist privilege for the federal courts (*Jaffee v. Redmond,* 1996). The case involved an effort by the estate of an individual who was killed by a police officer to obtain the records and testimony of a therapist who had seen the officer 50 times after the shooting. The trial court ordered the records produced and the therapist to testify. Both the therapist and the patient refused to comply. The jury then found for the estate of the decedent. However, the Supreme Court upheld a reversal of the trial court's order by the Court of Appeals, finding that both public and private interests would be served by protecting the privacy of clinical relationships from scrutiny in federal court proceedings. This case, because it relates to the Supreme Court's role in establishing the conditions under which the Federal Rules of Evidence are administered, may not have broader applicability to health information privacy issues. However, what is striking is the strong endorsement by the Supreme

Court for the need for confidentiality in the clinical relationship, even in the face of a plaintiff's claim that the information from that relationship was necessary to pursue a civil damages claim. In reaching its decision, the Supreme Court found not only a private interest in such a privilege, in order to facilitate the seeking of treatment, but also a public interest in the mental health of citizens, a public interest that the Supreme Court concluded would be furthered by insulating therapy from discovery.

Other Legal Issues Regarding Confidentiality

An individual who believes that his or her privacy has been invaded through an unauthorized disclosure of confidential health care information may bring a lawsuit under a number of theories. One theory is invasion of privacy, whereby a patient would claim that an unauthorized breach of confidentiality violated his or her right to privacy. A plaintiff might also claim breach of the clinician's fiduciary duty to the patient. As discussed previously, a clinician has ethical and legal responsibilities to patients, including a responsibility to honor confidentiality. A clinician who does not do so may be sued for breaching that fiduciary responsibility. If a contract between a provider and a payer creates an obligation to keep information confidential, then a patient could also claim that he or she is a third-party beneficiary of that contract and therefore entitled to recover damages for an unauthorized disclosure. Other theories include negligence; defamation, particularly if information disclosed about the patient is false; and negligent or intentional infliction of emotional distress, if the patient experiences mental injury from the disclosure. (A good discussion of these and related issues can be found in Hecker & Moses, 1994.) Although such lawsuits are rare, each theory is based on the ethical and legal duty of a mental health professional to keep information confidential unless the law permits disclosure.

PROBLEMS WITH THE LEGAL FRAMEWORK

As the preceding discussion suggests, there are many types and sources of confidentiality law. Some are quite detailed, others are cursory. Some are more protective of confidentiality than others. Some have been revised recently, whereas others have not been amended for some time. Some are probably quite adequate in providing to patients and clients reasonable assurances that information generated within the treatment relationship will not be disclosed inappropriately. However, in the aggregate, there are significant problems with the framework.

First, as noted previously, there is no national standard for the confidentiality of behavioral health records. There is a national standard for protection of the confidentiality of identifying information in the possession of federally assisted alcohol and substance abuse programs. However, that standard is significantly different from the standards established by most state mental health laws. In addition, the dual standards may create practical difficulties in determining whether and how to disclose information for providers who treat people who have co-occurring disorders.

Second, laws usually focus on information that is generated within the clinical relationship rather than on personal health care information in general. Most reform proposals would reorient legal rules to focus on what happens to personal health care information, regardless of who generates it or comes into possession of it.

Third, the access of families to information, particularly when the family is playing a caregiver role, is not consistent from state to state and is not permitted under federal substance abuse laws. As noted previously, this issue is not without controversy. However, a family's access depends entirely on the state in which the adult child is receiving care.

Fourth, there are significant differences among the states regarding when and under what circumstances information may be shared between providers. Most state laws have not been revised to acknowledge that multiprovider networks are the norm rather than the exception, so state laws often do not recognize the reality that the exchange of certain types of information between providers may be in the interest of client care as well as of cost containment.

Fifth, most state laws have not yet addressed the dramatic increase in the type and quantity of information demanded by payers of service. Many state laws permit the unauthorized release of information necessary to obtain payment. However, many of those laws were written in an era when a note or a summary was sufficient to gain payment. In addition, not all state laws regulate the use of information once it is acquired for reimbursement.

Sixth, many state laws do not differentiate between the types of information that are accumulated regarding an individual's mental health or substance abuse condition and treatment. Rather, most state laws are written in an "either/or" fashion: All information is available, or none is, depending on the circumstances governing disclosure.

Finally, most state laws do not acknowledge the complexity of the issue of consent to disclosure. For example, should individuals have the right to be informed of the manner in which a payment claim will be transmitted? If so, then should an individual have the right to deny consent to transmit the clinical information that must accompany the payment claim? Can the clinician deny treatment if the client will not give consent to disclosure because payment is unlikely to be forthcoming absent the underlying clinical information?

FEDERAL INITIATIVES

The problems with the legal rules that protect behavioral health care information also exist with the protection of general health care information. This has led many policy analysts and legislators to conclude that a national standard, created by the federal government, offers the only useful antidote.

Shapiro and Annas (1994) articulated core principles that might govern federal legislation. They argued that a national standard should define an individual's rights with respect to his or her health care information; define secondary users' legitimate access, rights, responsibilities, and prohibited uses; establish audit trails for all disclosures and requests for disclosures; prohibit redisclosure by authorized recipients as well as linkage to other data banks; establish medical record retention schedules; establish a unique identifier scheme used only for health care purposes; and establish oversight and enforcement mechanisms and a schedule of civil and criminal penalties for violations. Since the introduction of the Clinton health care reform bill in 1994, the move toward federal action has accelerated, a movement given additional stimulus by the HIPAA. Most proposals to create a national standard address the issues noted by Shapiro and Annas (1994).

The HIPAA contained several provisions addressing the privacy of health care information. It directed the Secretary of the DHHS to create "information guidelines" for health plans and providers. It also directed the Secretary to develop standards for the electronic transmission of health information (§§ 261–262). Finally, Congress directed the Secretary to report to it with recommendations regarding the privacy of "individually identifiable health information" (§ 264). The Secretary was to report on three topics: individual confidentiality rights, the procedures that should govern the exercise of such rights, and the uses and disclosures of information that should be authorized or required. The Secretary was to consult with the National Committee on Vital and Health Statistics, a committee established under the Public Health Services Act of 1974. Congress also directed the Secretary to promulgate regulations by February 2000 on the topic of health information privacy if Congress does not enact legislation by August 1999.

Congress, in enacting HIPAA, defined *individually identifiable health information* as

> Any information collected from an individual that (A) is created or received by a health care provider, health plan, employer, or health care clearinghouse; and (B) relates to the past, present, or future physical or mental health or condition of an individual, the provision of health care to an individual, or the past, present, or future payment for the provision of health care to an individual, and (i) identifies the individual; or (ii) with respect to which there is a reasonable basis to believe that the information can be used to identify the individual. (§ 262[6][A] and [B])

Although this definition does not bind Congress in the future, it may provide guidance regarding the definition that Congress might adopt in a national standard. Congress also directed that any federal regulation adopted by the Secretary under this statute not supersede any state law that is stricter than the federal rule (§ 264[c][2]).

The National Committee on Vital and Health Statistics (NCVHS) reported its preliminary recommendations to the Secretary of the DHHS Donna Shalala in July 1997, and the Secretary reported to the Congress in September 1997 (*Confidentiality of medical information,* 1997). Shalala's proposal joined a number of other legislative proposals that have been offered in recent years. Some of the most significant as of 1999 included those introduced by Senator Bennett (the Medical Records Confidentiality Act); Representative McDermott (the Medical Privacy in the Age of New Technologies Act); Representative Condit (the Fair Health Information Practices Act); and Senator Leahy (Medical Information Privacy and Security Act). The discussion that follows first describes the recommendations of the NCVHS and then discusses in general terms the issues addressed by the various reform proposals.

THE NATIONAL COMMITTEE ON VITAL AND HEALTH STATISTICS

The NCVHS was to recommend to the Secretary of the DHHS federal standards on the privacy of personal health care information. The NCVHS's Subcommittee on Privacy and Confidentiality assumed this task and in the course of its hearings heard testimony from many witnesses representing virtually all sectors of the health care industry.

In its June 25, 1997, recommendations to the Secretary of the DHHS, the NCVHS endorsed unanimously the need for federal legislation and urged Congress to enact a statute as rapidly as possible. In discussing possible legislation, the NCVHS recommended that health care information be defined broadly and include information generated and held by parties outside the clinical relationship. The NCVHS also urged the adoption of better technological protections for health records and stricter penalties for misuse of computer-based records.

On the issue of whether consent should be required for disclosures to payers of care, the NCVHS urged Congress to take a "real world" view but did not adopt a specific recommendation (R. Gellman, personal communication, November 25, 1997). The Committee did reject the argument that individuals should have the right to choose the technology used to create, store, and transmit individual health information.

The NCVHS supported broad researcher access to health records on the grounds that requiring patient consent would most likely result in stopping significant scientific research. The protections afforded by IRBs combined with strict penalties for abuse was considered adequate to protect individual privacy while permitting research to proceed. Broad access for public health purposes was also suggested.

Finally, the NCVHS recommended stronger controls to govern access to health care information by law enforcement officials, as well as stricter controls over the use of health care information by employers. The debate over access by law enforcement officials, as noted previously, is particularly contentious.

FEDERAL LEGISLATIVE PROPOSALS

The various legislative proposals placed before Congress in recent years, including Secretary Shalala's recommendations on behalf of the Clinton administration, generally are consistent with the philosophy of the NCVHS, though there are differences on substantive issues. The discussion that follows notes major points of agreement and contention in the debate regarding the creation of a national standard to protect the confidentiality of health care information.

Protected Health Information

An important element of all reform proposals is broadening the definition of information that is considered worth protecting. This is based on the assumption that health care information should include any information that identifies or could create a reasonable basis for identifying an individual and that is related to the past, present, or future physical or mental health or condition of the individual, the individual's treatment, or payment for treatment.

There is also agreement that organizations or individuals who come into possession of health care information should be obligated to protect the confidentiality of that information in much the same manner as health care professionals are. A term that some have used to describe those obligated to keep information confidential is *health care trustee.* There has not been complete agreement regarding how far the obligation to protect confidentiality should extend: All would cover health care providers and payers, but some question whether the obligation should cover school, employers, and others.

Consent Requirements

Another point of agreement is that a national standard should specify what constitutes a valid consent form. Most reform proposals would require that a consent form describe the information to be disclosed, describe the recipient of the disclosed information, provide the individual with the right to amend or revoke his or her consent, specify the purpose for which the disclosed information will be used, and provide a date at which the individual's consent expires.

An area of disagreement is when consent should be required or when it might be assumed. This issue is discussed in more detail in the next sections.

Access by Payers and Other Treatment Providers   A core question in the confidentiality debates is whether a provider of health care should be able to share information with other treatment providers and payers of health care without patient consent. Those who argue that consent should not be required often rest their argument on efficiency grounds: If a patient can prohibit information from flowing to other health care professionals and to payers, then care might suffer or the efficiencies that reimbursement systems presumably bring might be lost. Those who believe that the patient's consent must be required base their arguments on the values underlying confidentiality noted previously in this chapter.

Reform proposals as of 1999 have adopted one of three approaches to this issue. Some would require patient consent prior to virtually all disclosures to other providers and to payers (an exception would be the disclosure of information necessary to address a medical emergency). Proponents recognize that this might result in the denial of treatment to a patient—for example, if a health care provider concludes that he or she cannot adequately treat the individual in the absence of clinical information. It might also mean that an individual must pay for health care out of his or her resources because a payer would not be obligated to provide reimbursement in the absence of information.

A second group of proposals would permit disclosures of health care information without consent. A health care provider could still decide to obtain consent prior to disclosing information. However, these proposals would not require consent.

Finally, a third approach would assume consent but would permit the patient to "opt out" of specific disclosures. This approach, out of concern that traditional informed consent processes often give individuals little real choice, attempts to create a conversation between the practitioner and the patient regarding the specific types of disclosures that might occur. The patient could then direct that specified parties not receive information. Proponents of this approach recognize, much like the first approach, that an individual who does not consent to the release of information could forego treatment or third-party reimbursement as a result.

Disclosure to Law Enforcement Agencies   There are a variety of situations in which law enforcement officials might need to have access to health care information. These range from comparatively simple situations (an individual hospitalized involuntarily has left a hospital without permission and the hospital requests assistance from a police officer in finding and returning the person) to the extremely complex (health care fraud investigations presumably requiring access to records of hundreds or thousands of patients). The conditions under which access should be granted have been a matter of significant controversy (Hoge, 1995). As a general matter, most legislative proposals would permit law enforcement authorities to obtain access if they can show "probable cause" before a court that the information is relevant to a legitimate law enforcement inquiry being conducted by government authority. The recommendations of the Clinton administration sparked considerable controversy when introduced because they assumed that virtually complete access by law enforcement officials is necessary: "These disclosures are necessary to protect the health care system and the public, and they comport with certain well-accepted realities of law enforcement and the criminal justice system" (*Confidentiality of medical information,* 1997). It is likely that a national standard, if one emerges, will structure to at least some degree law enforcement access to health care information.

Emergency Disclosures   The previous discussion of state law notes that many states permit but do not require a health care professional to take steps, including the disclosure of confidential information, if he or she concludes that a third party might be at risk from the individual who is in treatment. Most reform proposals would codify this principle, permitting disclosure when 1) the subject of the disclosure is in danger and the disclosure is necessary to protect the subject's health or safety from serious harm and 2) when there is an identifiable threat of serious injury or death to an identifiable individual or group of individuals and the disclosure is necessary to prevent or significantly reduce the possibility of such a threat.

Access by Next of Kin   Most proposals would also provide some access to information by next of kin, an issue of interest particularly to family members of individuals with mental illness. Typically, health information regarding current treatment of someone on inpatient status could be provided to next of kin, an individual representative of the patient, or a person with whom the individual has a significant personal relationship, if the subject of the disclosure has been notified at the time of admission of a right to object to such disclosures and has not done so or if the subject is not in a condition to be notified. A provider could also refuse to disclose information if he or she concludes that disclosure would be harmful to the patient.

Access to Information by Researchers   The question of researcher access to information is an important one. In most states, researchers are obligated to obtain patient consent if the research involves potential risk to the individual or uses the individual as a direct source of information. In contrast, record-based research is often exempt as long as researchers do not reveal information that could identify an individual. Many proposals would continue to permit access to health care information without patient consent for record-based research if the IRB determines that it would be impracticable to conduct the research without such information and the anticipated benefit of the research outweighs the cost of the potential intrusion into individual privacy. At the same time, at least one proposal would require consent prior to the disclosure of any identifying information to researchers; disclosure without consent could occur only if the records were stripped of identifying information.

Audit and Oversight Activities   As a general rule, accrediting bodies and other oversight agencies have enjoyed broad access to health care information. There have been few suggestions that this situation should change. To the degree that reform proposals have addressed this topic, they have sought to ensure tighter control of information by oversight bodies once they obtain such information.

Public Health Activities   Another area in which broad disclosure generally has been permitted is for public health purposes. For example, information that permits the detection and tracking of infectious disease or the operation of disease registries traditionally has been disclosed to public health officials on the basis that the benefit derived from the protection of public health is more important than confidentiality. Most reform proposals endorse this approach.

Preemption of State and Federal Laws

An important question for behavioral health policy makers and treatment providers is the impact of a national standard on state mental health and federal substance abuse and alcohol laws. As noted previously, existing confidentiality law in the behavioral health field is a mixture of sometimes conflicting state and federal law. There are other diseases, most notably AIDS, for which state laws often create discrete confidentiality protections.

Most reform proposals adopt the principle that a national standard would create a "floor" for confidentiality. In other words, if a state had a more stringent protection in a particular area than the national standard, then the more stringent protection would prevail in the particular state. Otherwise, the national standard would govern. Some would assign to the Secretary of the DHHS the task of deciding whether particular federal laws addressing confidentiality (e.g., the substance abuse confidentiality law) are more protective and therefore should remain in place even after enactment of a national standard.

POLICY ISSUES FOR THE MENTAL HEALTH AND SUBSTANCE ABUSE FIELDS

There are a number of policy and legal issues that mental health and substance abuse policy makers, practitioners, families, and consumers/survivors should consider in determining the impact of a national standard on the confidentiality of mental health, substance abuse, and alcohol treatment information.

Preemption

Whether a national standard should replace all state laws is a complex but critical threshold issue. Most reform proposals would permit the states to retain stronger protections than those that would emerge in a national standard. Each proposal, in suggesting that states be permitted to retain stricter standards than a national standard if they so choose, uses mental health information as an example of a type of information often treated more protectively by the states. However, this assumption may be unfounded. In addressing the preemption of mental health and substance abuse laws, a number of questions need to be addressed:

1. Are state mental health laws, in fact, more protective than the various proposed federal standards? A review of state laws suggests that in many states, the answer to this question is "no." For example, all reform proposals would create standards for consent to disclosure, something absent in many state mental health laws. Each reform proposal also seeks to create a comprehensive statute; many state mental health confidentiality statutes have been enacted in piecemeal fashion, as issues arise.
2. What operational difficulties will arise in attempting to determine whether a particular state provision is more or less protective than the federal standard, a question that will dictate whether federal or state law applies? For example, if a state law permits unauthorized disclosures to providers but limits the types of providers that can receive such information, then is that state law more or less restrictive than a national standard that permits unauthorized disclosures to all providers but gives patients the right to opt out of specific disclosures? On the one hand, the state law is more restrictive because it limits the type of provider that can receive information without patient consent; on the other hand, the state law is less restrictive because it does not provide the patient with the opportunity to opt out of specific disclosures. This is a general problem with any legislation that sets a floor that states can exceed, but it may be a more pressing issue in the case of some state mental health statutes.
3. If the federal substance abuse laws are not preempted, does this represent good policy? None of the proposals under consideration would create a uniform standard for mental health and substance abuse information. Rather, each would leave largely intact the separate legal structures that exist. This is a significant issue, particularly given growing recognition of the prevalence of co-occurring disorders within the behavioral health care field.

In short, the assumption in many of the current proposals that state mental health laws are usually stronger than proposed federal standards may be erroneous. It is possible that this assumption, combined with a decision to leave federal substance abuse laws intact, could result in the creation of a national standard for general health care information, whereas mental health and substance abuse rules would continue to vary dramatically from state to state and between mental health and substance abuse providers within the same state.

Integrating Mental Health and Substance Abuse Standards

The federal substance abuse regulations rest on an assumption that a higher than usual degree of confidentiality is required to facilitate the provision of substance abuse treatment. Discrete laws for mental health confidentiality rest at least in part on the same assumption. However, as noted throughout this chapter, the substance abuse standards are considerably stricter than not only state health codes but also state mental health laws. This raises two questions. First, should mental health records and information receive the same protections as substance abuse treatment information? Second, if so, should substance abuse information (and, by extension, mental health information) continue to be treated more restrictively than other health care information, or should such information be addressed within a general privacy statute?

Substance abuse information originally was provided stringent protection because revelations of the conduct for which the individual sought treatment could result in criminal prosecution. Such a rationale does not typically exist in the context of mental health treatment, though issues of stigma and discrimination provided a persuasive rationale for affording mental health information discrete protection. However, providing different standards of protection is increasingly problematic, given the large number of people who have both a mental illness and a substance abuse diagnosis. It may be more logical to have one standard to govern both types of information, a resolution that could be reached by incorporating mental health information into the substance abuse rules or by providing mental health and substance abuse data with the same protection as general health care information.

The proposition that mental health and substance abuse information necessarily requires more protection than other health care information has been accepted but is largely untested empirically. More restrictive rules for each appear to rest primarily on an assumption that to be labeled mentally ill, an alcoholic, or a substance abuser is more stigmatizing and has more negative consequences for the individual than to receive a physical illness diagnosis. However, there is not clear consensus that certain diseases should be given more protection, and mental health and substance abuse consumers/survivors, family members, providers, and policy makers eventually may have to confront the argument that mental health and substance abuse information should be treated the same as general health care information under a national standard. One commentator argued that

> The creation of strict disease-specific standards so much restrains the dissemination of data in some systems that legitimate health goals are undermined, while other categories of data receive insufficient protection. Any argument that drug and alcohol abuse data deserve special protection rests on a weak foundation because many other health conditions raise similar issues of sensitivity and intimacy (e.g., HIV infection, STDs, genetic conditions, mental illnesses). (Gostin, 1996, pp. 503–504)

This is not to suggest that it is desirable to reduce the protections afforded substance abuse data, one possible outcome of consolidating substance abuse and mental health information within a general health care information law. However, it is worth considering whether there should be an integrated standard for protecting both substance abuse and mental health information. If this means creating a stricter standard for such information, objections can be anticipated; as noted, some experts on the privacy of health care information already dispute the wisdom of a health care information standard that permits differential treatment of certain types of information. However, not considering this question almost inevitably will leave in place a widely divergent and varied body of mental health and substance abuse confidentiality law.

Proposal of a Model Mental Health Confidentiality Statute

If policy makers conclude that decisions regarding mental health confidentiality should be left largely to the states and leave federal substance abuse laws intact, then should a model mental health confidentiality statute be proposed? As the previous discussion and the appendix on state laws at the end of the book illustrate, there is wide variety among the states in handling confidentiality and privacy issues. Although previous model statutes on confidentiality have not been widely adopted by the states,[2] a model mental health confidentiality law could be disseminated through the National As-

---

[2]Only two states have adopted a model statute titled the Uniform Health-Care Information Act created by the National Conference of Commissioners on Uniform State Laws in 1985. (Recommendations to the Secretary of the DHHS, pursuant to section 264 of the Health Insurance and Portability Act of 1996, § I B).

sociation of State Mental Health Program Directors, the National Alliance for the Mentally Ill and its state affiliates, and national and state consumer/survivor organizations. Although achieving consensus on all issues among these various groups would be difficult, a model statute at minimum might propose the following:

1. *Providing explicit criteria for consent forms signed by clients:* The federal substance abuse statute and regulations contain good examples of this. Consent forms could be limited to the specific disclosure contemplated rather than be a blanket disclosure.

2. *Creating limits on the information demanded by payers:* This would require amending the very general provisions in many state statutes that simply provide that information can be made available to payers. A model statute could at least limit disclosures to the minimum necessary for a payer to make a decision regarding payment and restrict use of information obtained by payers to prevent the sale or use of that information for marketing purposes. For example, notes detailing conversations between a patient and a therapist could be presumptively unavailable outside the treatment relationship.

3. *Ensuring the client access to his or her chart, with an opportunity to correct inaccuracies:* Some but not all state laws explicitly permit such access. Given the potential abuses of personal mental health information and the wide distribution of such information, a uniform right of access is a necessary and salutary development. Although such a right might not be unlimited—for example, in the case of information given by third parties in confidence—the underlying right should be part of all state laws if a national standard is not adopted.

4. *Ensuring access to certain types of information for families and/or others who are acting in the role of caregiver:* This is a potentially controversial issue. However, many families continue to act as caregivers for spouses, siblings, or adult children. It seems reasonable that families in that role receive the information minimally necessary to play the role—for example, information regarding medication and its effects and a description of the potential consequences of not taking prescribed medication. It should also be noted that all of the major proposals on health care information privacy have a provision for limited release of information to next of kin or significant others.

5. *Creating a uniform standard that third parties that are given access to information—for example, researchers, program evalua-*

tors, or quality assurance and license and certification staff—certify in writing that they will not make unauthorized disclosures of patient-identifying information: Most state laws contain a provision like this, but a model statute could provide language that strengthens the guarantee.

6. *Suggesting standards for access of law enforcement officials to mental health information that conceivably would place more limits on such access than that suggested by some of the current proposals:* The issue of access by law enforcement is a major issue in the debates regarding a national standard, and it may be that a model state statute would structure and restrict access to mental health records more than some of the federal proposals do.

7. *Suggesting standards for providing information to other providers:* State laws are quite varied on this issue and in many cases do not recognize that much care is provided by networks of providers. A model statute could suggest ways to structure the exchange of information among providers, perhaps drawing from one of the models presented by the federal proposals.

CONCLUSION

Few would disagree that there should be strong protections for the confidentiality of health care information, in general, and behavioral health care information, in particular. Individuals who seek treatment for mental illness or a substance abuse problem often do so at some risk of negative consequences if the fact or content of treatment is revealed.

At the same time, the existing legal framework that purportedly provides this protection varies dramatically from state to state and between state and federal governments. Many proposals to create a national standard would strengthen the statutory protections for general health care information. As this chapter suggests, the effect of a national standard on behavioral health information is less certain.

The questions that must be addressed in the future are important ones. Should autonomy in controlling information about one's health treatment and status ever yield to the desire to attain greater efficiencies in providing and paying for health care? Should families have access to information about a family member who is being treated for mental illness? Should researchers continue to have unimpeded access to health care records, or are the risks to privacy greater than has previously been assumed? Should there be special protections for mental health and substance abuse information?

Resolution of these issues will require continued attention to the values that underlie the ethical and legal principles of confidentiality. It will also require continued sensitivity to the fact that the motivation to seek treatment for diseases that continue to carry significant social stigma could be lessened if an individual cannot have some assurance of privacy. As the Supreme Court recognized in creating a federal psychotherapeutic privilege, such a development would have implications for individual as well as public health.

REFERENCES

American Medical Association, Council on Ethical and Judicial Affairs. (1997). *Code of medical ethics: Current opinions with annotations.* Chicago: American Medical Association.

American Psychological Association. (1992). *Ethical principles of psychologists and code of conduct* [On-line]. Available: http://www.apa.org/ethics/code.html

Barron, P., Goldstein, S., & Wishnev, K. (1995). State statutes dealing with HIV and AIDS: A comprehensive state-by-state summary. *Law and Sexuality: A Review of Lesbian and Gay Legal Issues, 5,* 1–512.

Confidentiality of medical information: Hearings before the Senate Committee on Labor and Human Resources, 105th Cong., 1st Sess. (1997) (testimony of D.E. Shalala, Secretary, U.S. Department of Health and Human Services, and Senator J. Jeffords).

Controlled Substance Act of 1970, PL 91-513, 21 U.S.C. § 801 *et seq.*

Dahm, L. (1997). Using the DNA profile as the unique patient identifier in the community health information network: Legal implications. *John Marshall Journal of Computer and Information Law, 15,* 227–275.

Donaldson, M., & Lohr, K.N. (Eds.). (1994). *Health data in the information age: Use, disclosure, and privacy.* Washington, DC: National Academy Press.

Fair Health Information Practices Act, H.R. 52, 105th Cong., 1st Sess. (1997).

Feenan, D. (1996). Common law access to medical records. *Modern Law Review, 59,* 101–110.

Freedom of Information Act of 1964, PL 89-554, 5 U.S.C. § 552(b).

Gostin, L. (1996). Health information privacy. *Cornell Law Review, 80,* 451–528.

Health Insurance Portability and Accountability Act of 1996, PL 104-191, 42 U.S.C. § 300(gg).

Hecker, S., & Moses, R. (1994, December). *Health plan confidentiality of information issues.* Paper presented at the National Health Lawyers Managed Care Law Institute: Legal and Structural Issues. Chicago.

Hoge, S. (1995). Proposed federal legislation jeopardizes patient privacy. *Bulletin of the Academy of Psychiatry and Law, 23,* 495–500.

Jaffee v. Redmond, 518 U.S. 1 (1996).

Lee v. Corregedore, 83 Hawaii 154, 925 P.2d 324 (Hawaii S.Ct. 1996).

Medical Information Privacy and Security Act, S. 1368, 105th Cong., 1st Sess. (1997).

Medical Privacy in the Age of New Technologies Act, H.R. 1815, 105th Cong., 1st Sess. (1997).

Medical Records Confidentiality Act, S. 1360, 104th Cong., 1st Sess. (1995).

Morgan v. Fairfield Family Counseling Center, 77 Ohio St. 284, 676 N.E.2d 534 (Ohio S.Ct. 1997).

Patterson, E. (1989). Health care choices and the constitution: Reconciling privacy and public health. *Rutgers Law Review, 42,* 1–91.

Peck, R. (1994). Results from an Equifax privacy poll: On concerns about medical confidentiality. *Medical and Health News, 14,* 10.

Petrila, J. (1992). Confidentiality and the family as caregiver. *Hospital and Community Psychiatry, 43,* 136–139.

Privacy Act of 1974, PL 93-579, 5 U.S.C. § 552(a).

Public Health Services Act of 1992, PL 102-321, 42 U.S.C. § 290(dd).

Schwartz, P. (1995). The protection of privacy in health care reform. *Vanderbilt Law Review, 48,* 295–347.

Shapiro, R., & Annas, G. (1994). Who sees your medical records? *Human Rights, 21,* 10–18.

State statutes or regulations expressly governing disclosure of fact that person has tested positive for human immunodeficiency virus (HIV) or acquired immunodeficiency syndrome (AIDS) [Annotation]. (1996). *American Law Reports, 12,* 149–193.

Tarasoff v. Regents of University of California, 551 P.2d 334 (1976).

T.C.A. 33-3-104(10) (LEXIS Supp. 1998).

U.S. Department of Health and Human Services, Center for Substance Abuse Treatment. (1994). *Technical assistance publication series: Confidentiality of patient records for alcohol and other drug treatment* (Number 13). Washington, DC: Author.

Whalen v. Roe, 429 U.S.589 (1977).

7

Will Technology Help or Hurt in the Struggle for Health Privacy?

Robert Gellman

INITIAL PERSPECTIVES ON PRIVACY

Technology and privacy have always been intertwined. The concept of a legal right to privacy was invented in the United States (Flaherty, 1989), at least partly in response to technological developments. The famous 1890 *Harvard Law Review* article that first proposed the right to privacy expressed concern about the new "instantaneous" photograph that allowed pictures to be taken surreptitiously and without a formal sitting (Brandeis & Warren, 1890). Now that live television coverage of criminal trials and video surveillance on public streets is routine, the fear of still photography seems refreshingly quaint.

Information technology has remained a constant theme in privacy discussions (Gellman, 1996a). In the 1960s and 1970s, public fears about government computers[1] contributed to the passage of the Privacy Act of 1974, which was the first law to regulate generally the use of personal information by federal agencies. Current privacy discussions center on the implications for privacy of computer networks such as the Internet (Federal Trade Commission, 1998). Encryption, smart cards, and biometric identifiers are examples of other forms of technology that have a significant effect on privacy interests.

---

[1]For a history of congressional activities on privacy during the 1960s and 1970s, see Regan (1995), pages 71–86.

Despite many years of debate, there is no consensus about the meaning and goals of privacy. Scholarly journals are filled with conflicting theories about the philosophy and purpose of privacy (see Regan, 1995). Perhaps because much of the development of the legal right to privacy has taken place in law journals, the confusion and lack of agreement may be entirely understandable. Privacy remains an issue of broad and almost unbounded dimension, encompassing everything from control over personal information to limits on government intrusion into the home to personal reproductive rights. Disputes extend to language as well as policy, and there is no agreement on the distinction between *privacy* and *confidentiality.*

The Europeans have a term—*data protection*—that is useful here (Bennett, 1992). Data protection focuses expressly on the collection, maintenance, use, and disclosure of personal information. Those are the principal concerns about personal records of all types, including health records. Although the term *privacy* is used in this chapter for convenience, it is intended to mean the same thing as *data protection.*

The policy content of modern privacy law is *fair information practices.* A code of fair information practices first was proposed in 1973 by an advisory committee at the Department of Health, Education and Welfare (Secretary's Advisory Committee on Automated Personal Data Systems, 1973). Similar principles were proposed at approximately the same time in England, and it is impossible to determine which came first (Bennett, 1992).

Later developments in Europe expanded that original concept. Since the late 1970s, virtually every privacy law enacted anywhere in the world is an implementation of fair information practices (Bennett, 1992; Council of Europe, 1981; Organization for Economic Cooperation and Development, 1980). Although no universally recognized code of fair information practices exists, most formulations contain the same elements.[2] Recognizing the importance of fair information practices, Representative Condit (D-CA) called his fed-

---

[2]One version of the code of fair information practices states the following:

1. *The Principle of Openness,* which provides that the existence of record-keeping systems and databanks containing data about individuals be publicly known, along with a description of main purpose and uses of the data.
2. *The Principle of Individual Participation,* which provides that each individual should have a right to see any data about him- or herself and to correct or remove any data that is not timely, accurate, relevant, or complete.

(continued)

eral health privacy bill proposal the Fair Health Information Practices Act.[3]

Fair information practices address the rights and responsibilities of record keepers and record subjects. Well-established legal principles are clear that the provider owns the document in which a patient's information appears. However, ownership is not important or even especially relevant to privacy. No matter who owns a health record—the provider, insurer, claims processor, or other health care institution—the patient clearly has an interest in how the information in that record is used, maintained, and disclosed. Ownership of a physical record does not and should not give the owner unlimited dominion over the data.

INITIAL PERSPECTIVES ON TECHNOLOGY

It is not necessary for the purposes of this chapter to define *technology*. It is important, however, not to overreact as the health care system integrates new forms of information technology. New technology creates both rational and irrational fears. Conversely, technological

---

3. *The Principle of Collection Limitation,* which provides that there should be limits to the collection of personal data; that data should be collected by lawful and fair means; and that data should be collected, when appropriate, with the knowledge or consent of the subject.
4. *The Principle of Data Quality,* which provides that personal data should be relevant to the purposes for which they are to be used and should be accurate, complete, and timely.
5. *The Principle of Use Limitation,* which provides that there must be limits to the internal uses of personal data and that the data should be used only for the purposes specified at the time of collection.
6. *The Principle of Disclosure Limitation,* which provides that personal data should not be communicated externally without the consent of the data subject or other legal authority.
7. *The Principle of Security,* which provides that personal data should be protected by reasonable security safeguards against such risks as loss, unauthorized access, destruction, use, modification, or disclosure. Sufficient resources should be available to offer reasonable assurances that security goals will be accomplished.
8. *The Principle of Accountability,* which provides that record keepers should be accountable for complying with fair information practices.
   (U.S. House of Representatives, Committee on Government Operations, 1994)

[3]H.R. 52, 105th Cong. (1997), introduced by Rep. Gary Condit (D-CA): "My legislation does not and cannot promise absolute privacy. What it does offer is a code of fair information practices for health information" (Congressional Record, 1997).

familiarity breeds acceptance, often far beyond what experience merits. Maintaining perspective is crucial.

Computers and computer networks are often described as sinister new threats to patient privacy. These concerns are real and cannot be dismissed. However, *paper* is a form of technology, and paper records have long been abused. Evidence comes from the only two detailed investigations into health record abuse conducted in North America in the last 30 years. Both took place in the late 1970s, long before the widespread use of computers.

In 1975, a Denver, Colorado, grand jury began an investigation into the theft of health records. It found that for more than 25 years, a private investigative reporting company engaged in a nationwide business of obtaining health information without patient consent. The company's investigators typically posed as doctors and sought information by telephone from public and private hospitals, clinics, and doctors' offices, including psychiatrists' offices. The company also paid hospital employees to smuggle health records. Another technique involved the use of false pretenses through mail solicitations. Customers for the information included more than 100 of the most prominent insurance companies in the country (Privacy Protection Study Commission, 1977; U.S. House of Representatives, Committee on Government Operations, 1980).

A 1980 report of an investigative commission in Ontario, Canada, offered even more spectacular evidence of abuse of paper-based health records (Royal Commission of Inquiry into the Confidentiality of Health Records in Ontario, 1980). The commission found that the acquisition of health information by private investigators without patient consent and through false pretenses was widespread. For the years 1976 and 1977, the commission documented hundreds of attempts to acquire patient information from hospitals and doctors in Ontario. Well over half of the attempts were successful.

So many insurance companies were using health information obtained under false pretenses that the Insurance Bureau of Canada made a *general admission* to the Royal Commission that its members had gathered medical information through various sources without the authorization of the patient. Many members of the Insurance Bureau of Canada were subsidiaries of American insurance companies, as were some investigative agencies that obtained information under false pretenses (U.S. House of Representatives, Committee on Government Operations, 1980).

Today, more health information resides on computers. As telemedicine services expand, the routine transfer for diagnostic and treatment purposes of health information across computer networks will also expand. Nevertheless, it will be a long time before the majority of paper health records migrates entirely onto computers. Whatever technology is used, however, it is a mistake to assume that records are necessarily better protected or at greater risk. Too many other factors, known and unknown, are involved. As is discussed in this chapter, computers offer new protections for privacy as well as new threats to privacy.

In both the Canadian and Colorado investigations, the principal investigators testified that, in their view, the practices that they discovered were widespread (U.S. House of Representatives, Committee on Government Operations, 1980). In neither case had anyone suspected the extent of the abuse prior to the investigation. One lesson to be drawn is that without an independent, rigorous investigation, it is impossible to say whether health (or other) records have effective privacy controls, whatever the storage medium.

Another distraction resulting from the focus on computers and networks is a misunderstanding of the source of threats to health record privacy. General discussions of computerized patient records invariably highlight the threat from outsiders who may break into computer systems and improperly obtain records. Although the threat from hackers is real, the more likely source of abuse is insiders who have a legitimate ability to obtain access for one purpose but who use records for unauthorized purposes.[4] A report on protecting electronic health information offers a balanced view of actual security threats and a taxonomy of threats by insiders, intruders, and outsiders (National Research Council, 1997).

Finally, people too often confuse privacy and security, thinking that better security will solve privacy concerns. Technological developments such as encryption can be especially distracting in privacy debates. Security, however, is just one component of fair information practices. Improved security will not provide patients with access to their records, resolve hard choices about who is entitled to

---

[4]"Security measures must protect against reasonably anticipated threats. The committee cautions, however, against treating security as simply the need to prevent hackers or outsiders from obtaining access to protected health information. That is only one element. There is evidence to support the belief that an equal or greater threat comes from misuse of information by those who have access to the information during the course of their routine activities. Insider abuse is a characteristic of virtually every computerized system containing personal information, and it may, in fact, constitute the greatest security threat" (U.S. House of Representatives, Committee on Government Operations, 1994, p. 107).

use health records, or make record keepers accountable for their actions. As important as security is, it is not a cure-all for privacy problems.

HEALTH RECORD PRIVACY PROBLEMS

To evaluate the consequences of technology for health privacy, it is appropriate to begin with an understanding of the current state of privacy protection. This is, unfortunately, a depressing starting point. Patients and their records have few legal protections. The National Committee on Vital and Health Statistics (NCVHS)—an advisory committee at the U.S. Department of Health and Human Services (DHHS)—offered recommendations on health privacy legislation. The NCVHS's principal findings and recommendations contained this gloomy assessment:

> The United States is in the midst of a health privacy crisis. The protection of health records has eroded significantly in the last two decades. Major contributing factors are ongoing institutional changes in the structure of the health care system and the lack of modern privacy legislation. Without a federal health privacy law, patient protections will continue to deteriorate in the future. (NCVHS, 1997)

A brief look at the specifics follows.

Uses and Users of Health Records

Patient information is the mother's milk of health care. In the routine course of treatment, payment, and oversight, dozens of institutions and hundreds of individuals may have access to and may redisclose the identifiable records of any patient. Few physicians and fewer patients are aware of the extent to which identifiable health information flows among the many organizations that participate in the health care delivery system.

In the United States, a third party usually pays for health care services (U.S. DHHS, 1995). The insurer who approves and pays bills is an integral participant in the physician–patient relationship and a principal recipient of health information. Because health insurance is a benefit commonly offered by employers, the insurer is often hired by the employer. This exposes more of the complexity of health data flows. Information created by providers is routinely disclosed to insurers and may also flow from employers to insurers and vice versa. Because federal and state governments provide or pay for much health care, they obtain large amounts of health data as well. All of these institutions—government, provider, insurer, employer—may play multiple roles simultaneously.

Intermediaries transfer claims data from providers to private and governmental insurers. A bill for services may move from a physician's office to a billing service to one or more clearinghouses and through one or more value-added networks before reaching the insurer (Gilligan, 1997). Bills for prescription drugs may have a parallel but separate path, moving from pharmacist to pharmacy benefit manager to insurer. Basic payment functions involve many separate entities. Information may flow in all directions between all entities.

Another reason for the routine sharing of information is the pressure to contain costs. Every institution that pays health bills struggles with rising costs. The growing for-profit health care sector also seeks increasing profitability.[5] In response to these pressures, providers, insurers, governments, and employers aggressively pursue cost-containment and utilization-review activities. The 1990s sparked tremendous growth of cost-containment strategies, including activities intended to ensure that the quality of care meets accepted standards. Examples are peer review, quality assurance, accreditation, and licensing.

Other information-intensive activities include auditing, fraud control, and law enforcement functions. The amount of fraud, waste, and abuse in the United States has been estimated to be 10% of all health care spending.[6] The dollar losses—measured in billions—are huge. Federal, state, and private entities work jointly and separately to combat the losses. Criminal investigations for fraudulent health care billing are routine and have become front-page news.[7]

---

[5]The value of patient information to support the marketing and sales of medical products and services (e.g., medications) has already become a factor in the restructuring of the health care industry. In one example, a pharmaceutical manufacturer (Merck) purchased a mail-order pharmacy (Medco). The purchase price reportedly was based in part on the value of the information in the databases of the pharmacy. Marketing uses of patient information are also increasing (O'Harrow, 1998).

[6]The General Accounting Office, the federal government's audit agency, regularly reports on aspects of health care fraud, waste, and abuse. The titles of recent reports are instructive: *Health Insurance: Vulnerable Payers Lose Billions to Fraud and Abuse* (GAO/HRD-92-69 [1992]); *Medicare: Antifraud Technology Offers Significant Opportunity to Reduce Health Care Fraud* (GAO/AIMD-95-77 [1995]); *Medicare Spending: Modern Management Strategies Needed to Curb Billions in Unnecessary Payments* (GAO/HEHS-95-210 [1995]); *Medicare: Millions Can Be Saved by Screening Claims for Overused Services* (GAO/HEHS-96-49 [1996]); *Health Care Fraud: Information-Sharing Proposals to Improve Enforcement Efforts* (GAO/GGD-96-101 [1996]).

The use of health data for clinical purposes creates other layers of data transfer. Treatment information routinely passes between physicians, hospitals, laboratories, and pharmacies. Each entity may maintain its own record-keeping system and may use its own contractors for computer, communications, legal, accounting, and other information-based services.

Finally, state and federal public health agencies routinely collect patient data. The tracking of communicable diseases is a traditional goal, but these agencies carry out many other activities, including treatment. Somewhat related are health research activities, which may be conducted by physicians, hospitals, public health authorities, academics, or private companies. Other data transfers are the result of the reporting of hospital discharge data to state agencies and of other health data to state, federal, private, and international disease registries.

This long list of health information users is not complete. The point, however, is clear enough. Many health care and other institutions obtain, use, disclose, and retain health records. In terms of the number of individuals and institutions with routine access to identifiable patient records, *patient records may be the most widely circulated of all personal records maintained by third-party record keepers.* It is difficult to maintain the myth that patient records are confidential.[8]

Lack of Legal Protections

No general federal statute regulates the privacy of health records.[9] The Privacy Act of 1974 applies fair information practices to health (and other personal) records maintained by federal agencies and some federal contractors. However, it does not cover most health

---

[7]Recent federal legislation illustrates congressional willingness to allow access to health records for criminal law enforcement purposes related to health care fraud. The Attorney General now has the authority to subpoena any health record. See the Health Insurance Portability and Accountability Act of 1996 (PL 104-191, §247; adding new §3486 to title 18, United States Code). The legislation also places some limitations on the use of subpoenaed records in actions directed against the subject of the records.

[8]"The principle of medical confidentiality described in medical codes of ethics and still believed by patients no longer exists" (Siegler, 1982, p. 1520). Siegler found that at least 25 and perhaps as many as 100 health professionals and administrative personnel had access to the records of an inpatient at a hospital.

[9]The Balanced Budget Act of 1997, enacted August 5, 1997, established the Medicare+Choice program and included a new confidentiality requirement for enrollees. Section 4001 of the act added new section 1852(h) to the Social Security Act:

(continued)

care providers, health care institutions, or health records. Other federal laws (38 U.S.C. §7332; [1994] 42 U.S.C. §290dd-2 [1994]) cover drug and alcohol abuse treatment records maintained by any institution that receives federal funds, but few health records fall under the protection of these laws. The absence of federal privacy protections for health records is not unusual. Generally, federal law covers very few important categories of personal information maintained by third-party record keepers (Schwartz & Reidenberg, 1996). The existence of a federal law that protects the privacy of video rental records only serves to underscore the capricious nature of federal statutory protections for privacy.[10]

We must look to state law to find privacy rules for most patient records. State laws, however, vary substantially in age, scope, and quality. Most states have dozens of uncoordinated laws that regulate some aspect of the collection, use, maintenance, or disclosure of health records. Some institutions and some records are covered by these laws, but large gaps in coverage remain. According to a survey of state laws, most but not all states impose a duty on physicians to maintain confidentiality. Fewer impose a similar requirement on other health care providers. Nine have confidentiality requirements for employers, and only four impose duties on insurers (Gostin, Lazzarini, & Flaherty, 1996).

Numerous reviews of health records law have reached the same conclusion about the inadequacy and incompleteness of state and federal health privacy laws. Words used to describe legal protections include *patchwork, gap, erratic,* and *morass* (Institute of Medicine, 1994; Office of Technology Assessment, 1993; Privacy Protection Study Commission, 1977; U.S. House of Representatives, Committee on Government Operations, 1980, 1994; Workgroup for Electronic Data Interchange, 1992). No one argues that the current legal

---

Insofar as a Medicare+Choice organization maintains medical records or other health information regarding enrollees under this part, the Medicare+Choice organization shall establish procedures—
(1) to safeguard the privacy of any individually identifiable enrollee information,
(2) to maintain such records and information in a manner that is accurate and timely, and
(3) to assure timely access of enrollees to such records and information.

This language has potentially broad applicability to health care providers, but it only covers a fraction of their records. Regardless of its scope, the language has little substantive content.

[10]The Video Privacy Protection Act, 18 U.S.C. §2710 (1994), was passed in 1988 following disclosure of the video rental records of Supreme Court nominee Robert Bork.

structure offers any consistent, uniform, or meaningful protections to patients.

Key Technology Issues

Technology will not provide a direct solution to the major privacy problems facing the American health care system. Technology will neither replace the need for health privacy legislation nor by itself reduce the value of or demand for health data. However, technology will provide partial or total solutions to some problems, will exacerbate others, and will create entirely new problems, all at the same time. Some elements of the code of fair information practices (e.g., security) clearly lend themselves to useful technological responses. Other parts of the code (e.g., access and correction rights) require policy decisions that could be implemented using information technology.

The rapid evolution of both technology and the health care system does not make evaluation of their intersection any easier. Nevertheless, it is possible to review some ongoing developments.

Standards and Administrative Simplification   The Health Insurance Portability and Accountability Act (HIPAA) of 1996 includes a major section on administrative simplification.[11] The stated purpose is to improve the efficiency and effectiveness of the health care system by encouraging the development of a health information system through the establishment of standards and requirements for the electronic transmission of health information (110 Stat. 2021, §261). Standardized administrative and financial transactions are less costly when conducted electronically rather than on paper. Savings estimates range in the billions of dollars (U.S. DHHS, n.d.).

The activities subject to administrative simplification include

- Enrolling an individual in a health plan
- Paying health insurance premiums
- Checking insurance eligibility
- Obtaining authorization to refer a patient to a specialist
- Filing a reimbursement claim for delivered health care
- Requesting additional information to support a claim
- Coordinating claims across different insurance companies
- Notifying a provider about payment of a claim

---

[11]HIPAA is sometimes referred to as *Kennedy-Kassebaum* or as *Kassebaum-Kennedy.*

These basic activities all involve the collection and disclosure of significant amounts of personal information.

Standardizing and computerizing these functions create large pools of identifiable health data in electronic formats. When administrative simplification was considered during the abortive Clinton administration health care reform effort, many observers thought that formal privacy protections must accompany the process. The HIPAA, however, includes only a few privacy provisions and leaves much of the work for the future.

HIPAA required the Secretary of the DHHS to submit detailed recommendations on privacy to the Congress by August 21, 1997 (U.S. DHHS, 1997). When preparing the regulations, the Secretary was required to consult with the NCVHS and with the Attorney General (110 Stat. 2034, §264[d]). If no privacy legislation has passed by August 21, 1999 (3 years from HIPAA's date of enactment), then the Secretary is authorized to promulgate privacy regulations within 6 months (110 Stat. 2033).[12]

However, the Secretary's authority to issue privacy regulations covers only electronic health care transactions, a subset of health information. This means that some health information would be regulated for privacy while identical information in another format would not. The Privacy and Confidentiality Subcommittee of NCVHS held a series of hearings on privacy in early 1997.[13] Most witnesses expressed a strong preference for privacy legislation over regulation.

The long-term privacy implications of HIPAA's administrative simplification requirements remain uncertain. The law is sure to speed up the computerization of health data that has already been under way. Congress may or may not meet its deadline of privacy legislation by August 1999. Failure to pass privacy legislation does

---

[12]HIPAA also includes two substantive privacy provisions. Section 262 adds a new section (42 U.S.C. §1177), which defines the wrongful disclosure of individually identifiable health information as a criminal offense. Although the goal of this section is appealing, the language fails to define what constitutes a wrongful disclosure. As a result, the criminal penalty has no immediate applicability to any specific behavior. Section 264(b)(2) establishes a policy that any federal privacy regulations shall not supersede a contrary provision of state law if the provision imposes requirements that are more stringent than the federal regulatory requirements. The precise meaning and application of this provision are unclear. It has the potential to allow state privacy rules to undermine the standardization otherwise required by HIPAA.

[13]The hearing dates were January 13 and 14 and February 4, 5, 19, and 20, 1997. Unedited transcripts from the hearings are available on the NCVHS web site: http://aspe.os.dhhs.gov/ncvhs.

not alter the timetable for health data standardization activities. They will continue regardless. Privacy regulations might fill some gaps, but it is difficult to assess how the Secretary of the DHHS might approach the regulatory authority. The job of preparing the regulations is certain to take much more time than the 6 months allotted in the law. It will be a difficult task with limited effect on the health privacy picture.

Another ongoing health record standardization activity that predates HIPAA is the effort to develop a computer-based patient record (CPR; Institute of Medicine, 1997). CPRs are intended not just to be an automated version of paper medical records but also to contain the entire scope of health information in all forms. Medical history, current medications, laboratory test results, x-rays, and other elements will be incorporated into the CPR of the future.[14]

The HIPAA standards activities and the CPR process are not directly connected, but there is considerable overlap between the issues and the supporters of both efforts. Everyone is aware of the privacy implications of the technical developments and of the need for specific health privacy legislation. HIPAA reflects an express decision that the United States should have electronic health information standards today and confidentiality legislation tomorrow (maybe). Both HIPAA and CPR may offer additional examples of how technology continues to forge ahead following its own timetable, regardless of the ability of privacy policies, laws, and regulations to keep pace.

Anonymized, Coded, and Encrypted Information   Of the many different users of health information, some have a clear need for fully identifiable data. Treatment and payment functions obviously require linking records with specific patients.[15] For other functions, however, the need for identifiable records may diminish or even disappear entirely. Some research, public health, cost-containment, oversight, and even law enforcement functions can be conducted in whole or in part without the need for patient identifiers.[16]

---

[14]For information on current activities, go to the web site of the Computer-based Patient Record Institute at http://www.cpri.org/.

[15]The health record system does a poor job of linking some patient records for treatment purposes. Over the course of a lifetime, an individual can easily have dozens of providers in locations around the country or the world. Those records are linked haphazardly, if at all, and treatment is less effective or more expensive as a result.

[16]At hearings held by the NCVHS Subcommittee on Privacy and Confidentiality, most nontreatment, nonpayment users indicated that at least some of their functions could be conducted using nonidentifiable data. However, no group of users said that nonidentifiable data would satisfy all of their needs.

If those who use health data for socially beneficial purposes can function without individual identifiers, then there is the prospect of a free lunch. Important activities can be completed without risk to the privacy interests of individual patients. Modern information technology can readily provide useful but nonidentifiable records. Although the goal is clear and the objective is worthy, the reality is not that simple.

First, deciding what constitutes nonidentifiable information is not always easy. Stripping names, addresses, and numbers from a record is not always enough to render it nonidentifiable (Sweeney, 1997). Non-unique data may be sufficient for someone with access to other personal data (e.g., driver's license) to link a seemingly anonymous record with a known individual. A description of a patient as a "bus driver with cancer" is not likely to allow anyone to identify the patient. Yet, if the physician offering the description comes from a small town with a handful of bus drivers, it is possible that someone will link the description with a particular bus driver known to have retired recently for health reasons. Similarly, many people would have no difficulty concluding from a description of a professional athlete with amyotrophic lateral sclerosis that the individual is Lou Gehrig.

Nonidentifiability is not an absolute attribute but a matter of degree. Two legislative proposals illustrate different legal standards for nonidentifiability. One, Medical Privacy in the Age of New Technologies Act, defines *nonidentifiable health information* as information from which it is impossible to ascertain identity and that cannot be linked or matched by a *foreseeable* method. This standard virtually requires a guarantee that data can never be linked under any circumstances. Meeting the standard clearly will be a challenge. Given the widespread availability of personal information from a multitude of public and private sources (Gellman, 1995) and the power of modern computers to sift data, the standard may be impossible to meet.[17] Furthermore, the proposed definition does not consider the possibility that information voluntarily disclosed by the

---

[17]The New York Statewide Planning and Research Cooperative System (SPARCS) collects information on patient encounters using an identification number composed of non-unique elements. The identification number consists of birthday (YYYYMMDD), last four digits of the social security number (SSN), first two characters of the last name, last two characters of the last name, first two characters of the first name, and gender (M/F). Anyone with access to a database of names, birth dates, and SSNs could easily match these identification numbers with individuals. This illustrates some of the difficulty of creating nonidentifiable records that are *impossible* to link with known individuals. Accuracy of matching for SPARCS is more than 99% but less than 100%.

record subject may permit identification or linking that would otherwise appear impossible.

The other bill, Fair Health Information Practices Act of 1997, approaches the issue by defining identifiable data. It defines *protected health information* to include data that identify the subject of the information or for which there is a *reasonable basis to believe* that the information can be used to identify the subject. Without a reasonable basis to believe that data can be linked to a particular individual, the data are not identifiable and not subject to statutory restriction. The *reasonable basis to believe* test used to distinguish between identifiable and nonidentifiable data is not as demanding as the test described in the first bill. (See generally Committee on National Statistics, 1993.[18]) More data will qualify as nonidentifiable. Other tests for nonidentifiability can easily be devised as well.[19]

Second, not everyone agrees that nonidentifiable data lack a privacy interest. The Medical Privacy in the Age of New Technologies Act of 1997 gives each individual the ability to veto the use of his or her information for the creation of nonidentifiable information. It is difficult to articulate what privacy interest remains if a record subject cannot be identified from a disclosure of nonidentifiable information.[20] Nevertheless, the proposal protects that interest.

---

[18]The Panel on Confidentiality and Data Access of the Committee on National Statistics recommended continued government work on this issue. The panel noted that zero-risk requirements for disclosure of statistical records were unrealistic and recommended a standard that calls for a "reasonably low risk of disclosure of individually identifiable data."

[19]Sweeney (1997) suggested that contractual arrangements between data users and data suppliers may be needed to control the way in which potentially identifiable data are used. This approach may work in many cases, but it may not be adequate if the goal is the production of public-use data tapes. Regardless, standardizing the rules that apply to disclosures of stripped health data is worth more exploration.

[20]This discussion does not specifically address the broader public policy question of balancing the sometimes competing values of health research, public health, cost containment, and so forth against personal interests in privacy. The Medical Privacy in the Age of New Technologies Act of 1997, with its more absolute protection for nonidentifiable uses of health data, appears to reject the need for balance. In its recent legislative recommendations to the Secretary of the DHHS, the NCVHS (1997) offered a different view about patient consent for research:

> The committee has no difficulty in taking a position on the thorny issue of researcher access to health records. The committee strongly supports the use of health records for health research. Identifiers should only be

(continued)

A restriction on disclosure of nonidentifiable data may create difficult dilemmas. Consider a psychiatrist who treats patients for depression with drugs. One patient objects to any disclosure of nonidentifiable data derived from his record. If the psychiatrist says in writing, at a public meeting, or even in casual conversation that she treats patients for depression with drugs, then the objecting patient may have a cause of action for breach of privacy. Even though it is impossible to distinguish one nonidentifiable patient from another, no one can say that the disclosure was not about the patient with the objection. Physicians may find it difficult to disclose even the most general descriptions of their practices or their patients. Statistical information about treatment successes and failures might be prohibited or useless. Even the classic medical comment, "There's a lot of that going around," might violate privacy rules if the disclosure of nonidentifiable data is restricted.

Third, coding offers techniques that permit more effective use of health records while offering protection for patient privacy interests. If identifiers are removed from records, then it may be impossible to tell whether two records relate to the same patient. When records from disparate sources are coded with a common coding scheme, however, then records can be linked over time and location. For the scheme to be effective, neither the code selected nor the information disclosed can be linked to an individual. For longitudinal studies and other forms of research activities, the linking of records can be essential to obtain useful results (for examples, see U.S. House of Representatives, Committee on Government Operations, 1980).

Coding, however, presents administrative challenges that go beyond the simple removal of identifiers. Codes could be assigned by a third party who receives the records, removes the identifiers, assigns the code, and passes the resulting coded data to the user. One sticking point is that a third party must be trusted to have access to

---

available when necessary, and there must be some independent review of research access. Institutional review boards provide one model for independent review. Patients must also be protected against the possibility that they will be identified through publication of research findings.

The committee recognizes the conflict between research and privacy, but requiring patient consent as a condition of researcher access is impractical and expensive. It would also most likely stop a significant amount of useful investigation. This is not in the health interest of individual patients or the general population. Patient privacy interests are adequately protected by independent review of research protocols, the earliest possible removal of identifiers, prohibitions against use of research records for actions against patients, and strict penalties against researchers who violate the rules.

the identifiable records and to safeguard the codes. One earlier legislative proposal, the Medical Records Confidentiality Act, permitted disclosures of identifiable data to intermediaries for the express purpose of creating nonidentifiable data for other uses. However, it appears that support for the creation of health data intermediaries has faded. The fear is that such intermediaries might become gigantic repositories for all health data.

Another approach is to develop a coding algorithm that permits the original record keeper to assign a code. When only one record keeper provides records, this is an easy task. As records are collected from more record keepers, it grows more difficult to apply a suitable coding scheme so that the resulting code (and the data attached to it) cannot be manipulated to reveal a patient identifier. Each originating record keeper would be responsible for maintaining the algorithm and the codes.[21]

Fourth, encryption offers broader security protections for identifiable records. Coding is a form of encryption, but the use of coding suggested previously is for a narrow purpose. Encryption offers security protections for entire records in a variety of contexts. This is especially important as health information becomes more digital and migrates to the Internet. Uses of encryption include providing user and computer authentication and access controls, protecting stored information and on-line communications against snooping and eavesdropping, validating information content against unauthorized modification, and validating the origin and content of transactions (National Research Council, 1997).

Encryption has the potential to be a powerful security tool, but it is not a cure-all for privacy problems and conflicts. Security measures that are based on encryption are still largely undeployed anywhere in public computing, let alone in health care (National Research Council, 1997). This will change over time, but it will not be easy or inexpensive. The task of employing encryption for the millions of daily health care transactions that take place in thousands of locations will require considerable policy, technical, and man-

---

[21]Other forms of coding or masking of information are possible as well. When a researcher needs general information about the age of a patient, it is possible to provide useful but inexact data. An actual birth date could be randomly shifted by plus or minus 30 days for each patient. Depending on the nature of the research, the same technique would work for admission dates and other data elements. This would make it much more difficult for anyone to identify a particular individual on the basis of other available information about that individual (see, e.g., Luft, 1997).

agerial resources. The administrative difficulties present a significant barrier.

Encryption should not be viewed as a complete solution for security. The report from the National Research Council (1997) noted that encryption transforms the access problem into a key management problem. When information has been properly encrypted, it is necessary to guard only the encryption keys and not the information itself. This should be a simpler task, but it is not a trivial one.

Encryption is not a complete solution for privacy anyway. Although encryption may prevent hackers and interlopers from obtaining usable health information, the greater problems of insider abuse of health care information remain. For any given health care record, hundreds of individuals in multiple organizations may have a legitimate need to obtain the information. By itself, encryption does not provide the rules that are necessary to distinguish between proper and improper uses or users. Encryption also does not ensure that those authorized to have access to the records will use the records only for legitimate purposes.

Fifth, despite the constraints and problems, the notion of using nonidentifiable records remains attractive. The specific tasks that support nonidentifiability—stripping identifiers, assigning codes, and encrypting data—obviously are much easier to do in a computerized environment. The same functions may take hours for a paper record with hundreds of pages, each with identifiers. As more records are computerized, it becomes possible to make greater use of nonidentifiable information to lower costs, improve quality, and make more health care available. This is the free lunch suggested previously.

Although computers bring benefits, they also bring new risks and new fears. Some risks are indisputably real. As more records are stored electronically, a security breach affects more people. A thief in a medical record room can carry or copy only so many physical records at a time. A hacker who enters a hospital computer system may be able to abscond with every patient record just as easily as one. As individual computer systems are linked and networked together, both the risks to privacy and the potential rewards to interlopers increase simultaneously (Institute of Medicine, 1994).

The fears about privacy and computers have produced several types of public and patient responses. A general misconception—one that has risen to the level of an urban myth—is that HIPAA mandates the creation of a central, national database of patient information. Nothing in HIPAA requires the creation of a national database, so the myth has no direct basis in law. However, with modern computer technology, the distinction between a single, centralized database and multiple, separately maintained but linkable databases grows dimmer every day. The myth may be legally incorrect, but there was an element of truth to it even before HIPAA was passed.

Another public response is an express rejection of computerization. Some patient and civil liberties advocates want each patient to be able to decide whether his or her record may be maintained on a computer or perhaps a networked computer (Haines, 1997), but it is not clear how far the choice should extend. Should patients be able to make choices about physician use of personal computers, networked computers, fax machines, or telephones (cordless, analog, digital, cell)?

Patient control over information technology is not a practical or desirable option. The NCVHS rejected it expressly.[22] However, even the limited demand is telling. The debate on this point underscores the urgency for adequate legal protections for health records, the need for effective security, and the importance of addressing public fears of computerized health records and health data networks. The development of even a small contingent of anti-computer patients is another reason that the potential free lunch from computerized records is not likely to be entirely free. Public acceptance of computerization cannot be assumed or taken for granted.

Unique Health Identifier   Privacy interests clash with the demands of the health care system for better identification methods for patients. HIPAA requires the Secretary of the DHHS to adopt standards for unique health identifiers for individuals, employers, plans, and providers (110 Stat. 2025, §262). Only the individual identifier requirement has generated privacy controversy.

The value of a patient identifier derives from the ability to link disparate records that are based solely on the identifier. With the many institutions that participate in health care and with so many

---

[22]"The Committee is not sympathetic to the notion that patients should have a choice in the technology used to create, store and transmit health information. This is not a choice that record subjects [have] for records maintained by other third party record keepers such as banks and employers. Requiring health record keepers—who are spending vast sums on computerization—to retain parallel paper systems is impractical and costly. It would deny the benefits and savings that the Congress has already determined will result from increased use of modern information technology. Computers are an inevitable part of modern health care and indeed are intrinsic to the actual delivery of hospital care today. Patients must accept this and move on to debate the proper protections for records in a computerized environment" (NCVHS, 1997).

routine, computerized exchanges of data, the ability to link records easily and with a high degree of assurance is attractive. Many health institutions use an identifier for this purpose, but no common identification scheme is in place. The social security number (SSN) comes the closest, but it is not universal.

It is impossible to find consensus on a patient identifier. The privacy community and substantial parts of the medical community are strongly against the use of the SSN.[23] They argue that the SSN is a poor identifier because it is not unique (more than one individual may use an SSN) and because it is not self-authenticating (e.g., no check digit). The major concern, however, is that the SSN is widely used for many purposes, and the SSN can be readily obtained from both public and private sources. As a result, use of the SSN allows easy matching of health records to other personal records and further undermines privacy. Others support the use of the SSN because it is already in widespread use and because it would be the least expensive identifier to implement. Some support use of the SSN with an additional check digit (Computer-based Patient Record Institute, 1997).

The selection of a patient identifier involves much more than choice of a number. It presents a complex and multifaceted mixture of privacy, policy, technology, and cost. The first problem is that the concern about linking health records with nonhealth records using an identifier is valid. Many major institutions play a role in providing, paying for, and overseeing health care. All would routinely have patient health identification numbers, including physicians, hospitals, pharmacies, dentists, labs, employers, insurers, public health authorities, nursing homes, government health agencies, schools, and others. A newly issued identification number limited expressly to health would still be available to many institutions.

It is not apparent that, as a practical matter, a health identifier could be controlled to avoid the possibility of other uses or unwanted data linkage. If a new health identifier were developed, someone would quickly develop a cross-reference between the new identifier and the SSN.

A second problem is that a high-quality, unique identifier would also be of great value for other purposes. The need for reli-

---

[23]The Internet community and large elements of the public are strongly opposed to any expanded use of SSNs, and the concern has a high emotional content. A controversy involving the availability of SSNs through Internet search services created a firestorm that resulted in a quick response from the Congress and a continuing investigation by the Federal Trade Commission (Gellman, 1996b).

able identification is common to many public and private activities. There would be enormous political pressure to allow a new health identifier to be used for government programs such as welfare, motor vehicle licensing, debt collection, child support enforcement, and immigration control. Legislation could, in theory, deny use of a health identifier for these other purposes. In practice, however, it is unlikely that the Congress could resist allowing use of the new number for politically popular purposes. The SSN originally was intended to be used only for social security pensions. Over the years, Congress specifically authorized its use for tax, military, welfare, drivers, draft registration, and many other purposes.[24] A legislative attempt to restrict use of a health number likely would fail, either initially or eventually.

A third problem is that society is on the verge of a new era of identification technology. New options, including digital signatures and public key encryption, may be just around the corner (National Research Council, 1996). The main identification choices proposed as of 1999 are based mostly on old technology. The SSN itself is the Model-T of identification systems. Even with the addition of a check digit, it is no more advanced than a '57 Chevy. Until new alternatives are developed and tested, selection of an identifier may be premature. A choice made in haste today could easily become obsolete in a few years.

A fourth problem is that a unique patient identifier may be unnecessary to link records. Work is under way on a *master patient access mediator,* which will mediate linkage between health records systems with disparate patient identifiers (Lorton, 1997). Billions of existing health records include no identifier, so the problem of linking legacy records will continue no matter which new identifier is selected. The mediator would allow matching of old and new records without a common identifier.[25]

One of the strongest objections to an identifier is its ability to support record linkage. If linkage is possible anyway without an identifier, then we may be damned if we have one and damned if we don't. If comprehensive legislation effectively restricted the use and disclosure of health records, concern about the identifier and about linkage might even fade.

As the public debate on the health identifier issue began in earnest in 1998, another factor in the decision-making process emerged. Significant public opposition to a health identifier devel-

---

[24]See, for example, 42 U.S.C. 405(c)(2)(C)(i) (1994).

[25]For more information on efforts to establish master patient indices, go to http://www.acl.lanl.gov/cpr/.

oped as the NCVHS started the hearing process. Intense media coverage of the issue helped to elicit a political reaction, and legislative proposals that would stop the development or deployment of a patient identifier quickly emerged. The vice president issued a statement on July 31, 1998, indicating that the Clinton administration would not implement a patient identifier until statutory privacy protections were in place.

Identifiers and data linkage are issues whereby technological developments may ultimately make a difficult policy choice unnecessary or may reduce the stakes involved in the choice. There will always be some value in linking together all records about a single patient. Using a single patient identifier to accomplish data linkage may be an idea whose time has already passed. Regardless, technology alone will not determine whether protections for patients are improved or reduced as a result of a decision about an identifier. Legislation or restructuring of the health care system will play a much greater role. Public opinion may be an important factor as well.

NATIONAL VERSUS STATE VERSUS INDIVIDUAL PRIVACY POLICIES

Some of the most difficult health information policy choices involve the proper level of privacy regulation. The broadest issue is whether a federal health privacy law should preempt state laws. Among significant portions of the health care establishment, the demand for federal preemption and for a single national privacy standard is strong. The interstate nature of health care treatment and payment as well as HIPAA argue for uniformity. Growing telemedicine activities only underscore the problem of complying with multiple state laws.

The counter argument is that state laws that are more protective of privacy should be allowed to prevail over a weaker federal law.[26] HIPAA is inconsistent on this point and can be cited in support of both national standards *and* preserving stronger state privacy laws. The NCVHS (1997) legislative recommendations described preemption as "perhaps the most difficult conflict."

A second and related issue is whether all health information should be governed by uniform privacy standards or some health data should be viewed as more "sensitive" and subject to special

---

[26]The relative strength of state health privacy laws and the yet-to-pass federal law is impossible to assess. However, few existing state laws offer general privacy protections that match or exceed any of the proposed federal bills. Some narrowly focused state laws, such as AIDS laws, may have some protections that compare favorably with federal proposals.

rules. Existing laws at the state and federal levels already provide separate rules for records about alcohol and drug abuse, AIDS, genetic tests, and psychiatric conditions. The precedent for separate treatment is clear, but the practicality of supporting multiple privacy rules for different types of information in the same record is challenging at best.[27] An alternative approach is to afford all records the same "high level" of protection. A common rule would be much easier administratively and would avoid the need to rank health conditions based on the perceived sensitivity of a diagnosis or treatment.

The debate about these issues has taken place at a high level of generality. Interest groups have tended to identify themselves as for or against preemption or uniformity. This may be too simplistic. The NCVHS (1997) suggested breaking down some of these issues into their components and analyzing them separately.

Technology ultimately may offer a way of helping to address the practicality and the cost of diverse rules across states or within records. As discussed previously, computers allow health records to be more readily anonymized or coded so that they can be used for socially beneficial purposes without affecting individual privacy interests. The possibility that computers may be useful in addressing preemption or uniformity has not been explored. The ability of computers to manage different policies for different patients suggests that at least some policies might be tailored to individual preferences. Patient choice may be a possible level of regulation beyond that of federal or state law.

The principal arguments for federal preemption are standardization and cost. The prospect of complying with 50 different state laws is daunting in the interstate health care system. However, it is almost certainly unavoidable, even under the most preemptive of federal proposals. For example, no one has proposed allowing a federal health privacy bill to alter the diversity of state public health reporting statutes. Each state surely will continue to have its own requirements. A health care information computer system that supports treatment in more than one state must be programmed to comply with the reporting requirements of each relevant state. Similarly, no federal bill has proposed to substitute a nationwide rule on rights of minors. The bills that address rights of minors (e.g., Fair Health Information Practices Act) defer to state law on key issues.

---

[27]Distinguishing between different categories of information is challenging as well. Consider the case of a drug abuser suffering from AIDS and depression who has been identified as having a genetic predisposition to drug abuse. Identifying which data elements would be subject to which rules (drug abuse, AIDS, psychiatric, genetic, or "regular") is not a simple task.

Institutions that operate on a nationwide basis will be obliged to comply with state laws in these and other instances. Once it is accepted that computerized systems must account for the diversity of state laws, what remains is the relatively simpler task of programming for the alternatives. A harder task is to identify and resolve direct conflicts between state laws and to develop rules in cases in which state laws overlap.

It is important to identify those areas when a diversity of state law can be readily and cost-effectively accommodated by existing or future health information computer systems. The policy conflict between federal preemption and state laws might be partially resolved by using technology as one mediator. A preliminary question in each case is whether the diversity can be practically managed by existing or future health record management systems. Diversity that is difficult in a paper environment may be supportable in a computerized one.

Even if technologically possible, diversity will not work for policy reasons in some areas. The federal government is likely to insist on a uniform right of access to health records for federal oversight activities despite any contrary state interests. In other cases, no point may be served by allowing states to have their own rules. For instance, allowing 50 separate first-party access procedures might be unnecessarily expensive, yet some states with patient access laws entitle a patient to a free copy of his or her records. Others permit a charge for a copy. That policy difference may well be worth preserving.

Two broad principles for evaluating whether diversity is supportable are cost and the effect on interstate activities. If the cost of diversity is too great, then it would be reasonable to disallow the option. Similarly, one might reject a state policy that undermines technical or other standards necessary for efficient flow of electronic health transactions. An example is the type of encryption used for networked health transactions. If each state insisted on a different encryption technology or key length, then it could be impossible to use encryption for interstate transactions.

An analysis of policies for uniformity might proceed along similar lines. It seems unlikely that all existing laws for specific classes of health information would be superseded by any federal health privacy bill. For example, none of the existing proposals eliminates state AIDS laws or the federal alcohol and drug abuse laws. This means that a general federal law must coexist with some other laws.

Two key constraints can be identified. The first is the administrative burden of having two (or more) different laws apply to the records of the same patient. With a properly designed computerized health information system, this may be possible.[28] The second constraint is the difficulty of categorizing classes of records. For example, the line between genetic and mental health records may be clear today; tomorrow's discovery of a new genetic component to a psychiatric disorder could easily blur the categories. This is not a trivial concern.

A procedural method for assessing whether a particular limitation could be tolerated is to allow the Secretary of the DHHS to make the assessment under a statutory standard. Any state law that offers useful privacy protections and that is not unduly burdensome to record keepers could be allowed to stand if it does not interfere with the basic interstate flow of transaction information.[29] Assessing current and expected technological capabilities of computer and network health data management systems could be part of the Secretary's responsibility. Tying the decision to technology would allow for the result to change as technology improves.

Finally, technology may support a greater degree of patient control of health information. A precedent for greater consumer choice in the use of personal records is the Drivers Privacy Protection Act.[30] This federal law requires states to offer a choice to each driver before making some personal information available for disclosures for specified purposes including marketing. For other types of disclosures, the individual has no choice because disclosure is mandated or permitted by state or federal law.

This model may work for some disclosures of health information. Patients are not likely to be allowed a choice about some types

---

[28]A controversy that arose in Boston in 1996 illustrates how computers can manage different rules for different types of health records when the records can be clearly defined. Harvard Pilgrim Health Care's policy of making full records available on its computer system came under attack. In response, information about mental health treatment was restricted in availability on the computer system. This case raises medical questions about how widely patient records should be available to treating physicians. For example, when does an emergency room physician need to have access to the treatment notes of a psychiatric patient? Medical issues of this type are beyond the scope of this chapter, but technology may support the ability to allow patients to make some of these judgments and accept the consequences thereof.

[29]A somewhat similar concept is employed in the Fair Health Information Practices Act of 1997. Conflicts between a general federal privacy law and existing alcohol and drug abuse statutes would be resolved by directing the Secretary of the DHHS and the Secretary of Veterans Affairs to determine by regulation which provision provides greater privacy protection.

[30]18 U.S.C. §§2721–2725 (1994). The constitutionality of portions of the drivers privacy law has been called into question, but the constitutional uncertainties are not relevant to the analyses here.

of nonconsensual disclosures. Congress is likely to insist that records be available for fraud and abuse investigations, some law enforcement activities, and public health purposes. Patient consent may be possible or appropriate for other disclosures. At least one state requires patient consent for research disclosures (Minn. Stat. § 144.335 Subd. 3a[d] [Supp. 1997]). Whether this is a desirable result is an open question,[31] but the law shows that the patient choice model has some political support. Existing proposals also allow patients to veto specific disclosures to next of kin or of directory information.[32] By recognizing that patient choice is sure to be a factor in some disclosure (and perhaps other) decisions, computer systems can be designed to accommodate it. The result could be an inexpensive method of allowing for patient control over some uses and disclosures of patient records.

Physicians often act as advocates for patient privacy interests and exercise choices that their patients might desire, expect, or request. One way physicians prevent disclosure of patient information is to avoid writing it down. Another way is to maintain a separate, personal, and unofficial record as an adjunct to the official record. Mental health treatment notes are a classic example. These notes may be maintained in an entirely separate filing system and not routinely disclosed to anyone. In principle, technology can support unofficial records or can even assign confidentiality rankings to individual data elements.

Although computerized systems can accommodate tiers of confidentiality,[33] this capability may not really help. Once unofficial

---

[31]NCVHS (1997) rejected patient consent for research as impractical and expensive and as a barrier to significant investigation.

[32]The Medical Privacy in the Age of New Technologies Act allows patients to designate any part of their record as a *protected health information subfile.* Subfiles would be subject to narrower rules on use and disclosure. This may not offer an effective model, however, because patients and their providers would have a clear incentive to designate all records as protected subfiles. If the health care system can function under the more restrictive use and disclosure rules, then there is no reason to have more liberal rules for some records. If the restrictive rules interfere with other necessary functions, however, then the *subfile* approach is flawed.

[33]Where records are maintained in a filing system (computerized or otherwise) that is not under the personal control of the physician, even formally recognized unofficial records may be released by the proprietor of the system. Protections against this are possible. For example, a physician may encrypt sensitive patient notes so that the notes are unintelligible to all but the physician. This is risky business. The loss of the physician's encryption key could make the note completely irretrievable. Escrowing of keys is a protection against their loss, but this undermines the confidentiality being sought. Regardless of who controls the key, a subpoena can mandate the decrypting of records, and nonpayment of bills can provide an almost equally powerful incentive.

records are officially recognized and supported, users of the records, such as payers and fraud investigators, may well demand access. Payers can easily obtain patient consent for access with the threat of nonpayment, and law enforcement agencies can use compulsory process for the records. Conflicts over who can use records will not be avoided by special designations within computer systems. If anything, conflicts may be sharpened because the existence of the records is known.

Unless guarantees can be provided that some records are not available for any purpose at all—and this seems highly unlikely—the formal recognition of unofficial records may not offer any new protection for privacy interests. The result might only be to drive a physician's personal notes even further underground.

In each of these cases—preemption, uniformity, and patient/physician choice—well-designed computer systems can play a role in resolving or minimizing policy conflicts. The result can be better and more precise privacy policies that meet individual requirements. Technology offers useful capabilities that will enhance privacy, but it will offer only an occasional solution to the difficult policy choices that are unavoidable with the modern health care system.

Further, for technology to work in a more fully computerized environment, system designers must know in advance the requirements. Once accomplished, implementation of choices may be simple compared with managing multiple alternatives with paper records. Given the lengthy life cycle of computer systems, however, it could take many years before the technical support for a diversified policy could be in place nationwide. Solutions based on technological capabilities may have to be phased in slowly to allow time for new technology to become widespread.

CONCLUSION

The question posed in this chapter is whether technology will help or hurt in the struggle for health privacy. The answer is surely *yes.* Technology will both help and hurt. More widespread use of computers and networks will threaten privacy because patient information may be more readily available to more users. At the same time, the technology may improve patient care and lower costs. Computers may also enable us to manage patient information so that we can profit from its availability in ways that do not impinge further on individual privacy interests. Well-managed computer systems can also provide greater security protections. All of this can be done, but it remains to be seen whether they will be done in a safe and effective way.

Technology moves relentlessly ahead. With each advance, health system participants (and vendors) see the benefits and press for implementation of new options. Up to a point, legislative support for technology is not required. In any event, HIPAA provides a basis for coordinating many health information technological developments for the immediate future.

The same political support for privacy regulation has been missing. Institutional and technological activities can do much to protect privacy interests of patients, but they cannot solve most of the existing legal and policy shortcomings. Whether the political will to pass privacy legislation can be found is open to question. Future prospects for legislation remain highly uncertain.

The biggest danger from ever-expanding uses of technology may come from the way that they affect existing constitutional standards about privacy. In interpreting the Fourth Amendment's protections against unreasonable searches and seizures, the Supreme Court looks in part at the expectations of individuals and society.[34] This test is tautological. Privacy is protected only when people expect it to be protected. As Professor Paul Schwartz has written, "This circular approach ignores the silent ability of technology to erode our expectations of privacy" (1995, p. 553).

It remains to be seen whether the growing gap between privacy and technology will create a consumer backlash or the requisite pressure for legislation. Evidence of a backlash exists, but it does not appear to pose either a real threat to computerization or a sufficient force to drive legislation through the Congress.

It was stated previously in this chapter that technological familiarity breeds acceptance. But it may be far worse than that. Familiarity may change the way in which the privacy implications of technology are evaluated constitutionally. Once everyone is used to technology, it grows more difficult to argue that the technology violates expectations of privacy. The only protections will be those that are legislated.

Because of the central role that technology will play in the processing and maintenance of patient records, it will always be impor-

---

[34]The Fourth Amendment protects only against governmental actions. It does not protect against actions by private parties. In a leading case on a constitutional right of information privacy involving health information, the Supreme Court declined the opportunity to find that the right existed. In *Whalen v. Roe* (1976), the court held that if such a right existed, it was not violated in that case.

tant in decisions about privacy protections. Technology, however, is only a tool. The key health privacy concerns identified in this chapter are the widespread use of identifiable health information and the lack of adequate legal protection. Technology cannot address the basic policy choices about which institutions should be permitted to use identifiable records for which purposes and what kind of laws are needed. To be sure, technology will help to shape the responses to these questions. Yet technology is not the only answer. The difficult tradeoffs among privacy, efficiency, quality, and cost must be confronted and resolved. Progress on the health privacy front will remain limited without new federal legislative protections.

REFERENCES

Bennett, C. (1992). *Regulating privacy: Data protection and public policy in Europe and the United States.* Ithaca, NY: Cornell University Press.

Brandeis, L., & Warren, S. (1890). The right to privacy. *Harvard Law Review, 5,* 193–220.

Committee on National Statistics. (1993). *Private lives and public policies: Confidentiality and accessibility of government statistics.* Washington, DC: National Research Council.

Computer-based Patient Record Institute. (1997). *Annual report.* Bethesda, MD: Author.

Council of Europe. (1981). *Convention for the Protection of Individuals with Regard to Automatic Processing of Personal Data.* European Treaties, ETS No. 108, Strasbourg, 28.I.1981.

Drivers Privacy Protection Act of 1994, PL 103-322, 18 U.S.C. §§ 2721–2725.

Fair Health Information Practices Act of 1997, H.R. 52, 105th Cong., 1st Sess. (1997).

Federal Trade Commission. (1998). *Privacy online: A report to Congress* [On-line]. Available: http://www.ftc.gov/reports/privacy3/toc.htm

Flaherty, D. (1989). *Protecting privacy in surveillance societies.* Chapel Hill: University of North Carolina Press.

Gellman, R. (1995). Public records—Access, privacy, and public policy: A discussion paper. *Government Information Quarterly, 12,* 391.

Gellman, R. (1996a). Can privacy be regulated effectively on a national level? Thoughts on the possible need for international privacy rules. *Villanova Law Review, 41,* 129–172.

Gellman R. (1996b, November 18). 2 Studies—1 Fed, 1 FTC—Focus on net privacy. *DM News,* p. 18.

Gilligan, T. (Executive Director, Association for Electronic Health Care Transactions). (1997, February 4). Testimony before the National Committee on Vital and Health Statistics [On-line]. Available: http://aspe.os.dhhs.gov/ncvhs/970204tr.htm

Gostin, L., Lazzarini, Z., & Flaherty, K. (1996). *Legislative survey of state confidentiality laws, with specific emphasis on HIV and immunization.* Presented to the U.S. Centers for Disease Control and Prevention [On-line]. Available: http://www.epic.org/privacy/medical/cdcsurvey.html

Haines, D. (American Civil Liberties Union). (1997, February 19). Testimony before the Subcommittee on Privacy and Confidentiality, National Committee on Vital and Health Statistics [On-line]. Available: http://aspe.os.dhhs.gov/ncvhs/970219tr.htm

Health Insurance Portability and Accountability Act of 1996, PL 104-191, 42 U.S.C.

Institute of Medicine. (1994). *Health data in the information age: Use, disclosure, and privacy.* Washington, DC: National Academy Press.

Institute of Medicine. (1997). *The computer-based patient record.* Washington, DC: National Academy Press.

Lorton, L. (Executive Director, Health Care Open Systems and Trials). (1997, February 18). Testimony before the Subcommittee on Privacy and Confidentiality, National Committee on Vital and Health Statistics [On-line]. Available: http://aspe.os.dhhs.gov/ncvhs/970219tr.htm

Luft, H. (Professor of Health Policy and Health Economics, University of California, San Francisco). (1997, June 3). Testimony before the National Committee on Vital and Health Statistics [On-line]. Available: http://aspe.os.dhhs.gov/ncvhs/970603tb.htm

Medical Privacy in the Age of New Technologies Act of 1997, H.R. 1815, 105th Cong., 1st Sess. (1997).

Medical Records Confidentiality Act, S. 1360, 104th Cong., 1st Sess. (1995).

National Committee on Vital and Health Statistics. (1997). Health privacy and confidentiality recommendations [On-line]. Available: http://aspe.os.dhhs.gov/ncvhs/privrecs.htm

National Research Council. (1996). *Cryptography's role in securing the information society.* Washington, DC: National Academy Press.

National Research Council. (1997). *For the record: Protecting electronic health information.* Washington, DC: National Academy Press.

Office of Technology Assessment. (1993). *Protecting privacy in computerized medical information.* Washington, DC: Government Printing Office.

O'Harrow, R. (1998, February 15). Prescription sales, privacy fears CVS, Giant share customer records with drug marketing firm. *The Washington Post,* p. A1.

Organization for Economic Cooperation and Development. (1980). Council Recommendations Concerning Guidelines Governing the Protection of Privacy and Transborder Flows of Personal Data. 20 I.L.M. 422 (1981), O.E.C.D. Doc. C (80) 58 (Final) (Oct. 1, 1980).

Privacy Act of 1974, PL 93-579, 5 U.S.C. § 552a.

Privacy of Medical Information Act, H.R. 5935, 96th Cong., 1st Sess. (1979).

Privacy Protection Study Commission. (1977). *Personal privacy in an information society.* Washington, DC: Government Printing Office.

Regan, P. (1995). *Legislating privacy.* Chapel Hill: University of North Carolina Press.

Royal Commission of Inquiry into the Confidentiality of Health Records in Ontario. (1980). *Report of the Commission of Inquiry into the Confidentiality of Health Information.* Ontario, Canada: J.B. Thatcher.

Schwartz, P. (1995). Privacy and participation: Personal information and public sector regulation in the United States. *Iowa Law Review, 80,* 553–618.

Schwartz, P., & Reidenberg, J. (1996). *Data privacy law.* Charlottesville, VA: Michie.

Secretary's Advisory Committee on Automated Personal Data Systems. (1973). *Records, computers, and the rights of citizens.* Washington, DC: U.S. Department of Health, Education & Welfare.

Siegler, M. (1982, December 9). Confidentiality in medicine—A decrepit concept. *New England Journal of Medicine, 307,* 1518–1521.

Sweeney, L. (1997). *Maintaining patient confidentiality when sharing medical data requires a symbiotic relationship between technology and policy* (Working Paper No. AIWP-WP344b). MIT Artificial Intelligence Laboratory.

U.S. Department of Health and Human Services. (1995). *Health United States 1994.* Washington, DC: Government Printing Office.

U.S. Department of Health and Human Services. (1997). *Confidentiality of individually-identifiable health information* [On-line]. Available: http:// aspe.os.dhhs.gov/admnsimp/pvcrec0.htm

U.S. Department of Health and Human Services. (n.d.). *Health Insurance Portability and Accountability Act of 1996: HHS implementation of administrative simplification requirements* [On-line]. Available: http:// aspe.os.dhhs.gov/datacncl/kkimpl.htm

U.S. House of Representatives, Committee on Government Operations. (1980). *Federal Privacy of Medical Information Act.* H.R. Rep. No. 832, Pt. I (report to accompany H.R. 5935).

U.S. House of Representatives, Committee on Government Operations. (1994). *Health Security Act.* H.R. Rep. No. 601, pt. 5, 103rd Cong. 83 (report to accompany H.R. 3600).

Video Privacy Protection Act of 1988, PL 103-322, 18 U.S.C. § 2710.

Whalen v. Roe, 429 U.S. 589 (1976).

Workgroup for Electronic Data Interchange. (1992). *Report to Secretary of U.S. Department of Health and Human Services.*

8

Confidentiality and HIV/AIDS
Professional Challenges

Robert L. Barret

Prior to the 1980s, the mental health community's debate about confidentiality took place in somewhat predictable domains. Issues of medical records, threats of harm to self or others, and many of the topics covered in other chapters in this book framed the context of the discussion. The advent of HIV in the early 1980s extended this debate into new territory and has raised questions about the limits of confidentiality that remain unanswered. Psychologists, social workers, counselors, and other mental health professionals found themselves sitting with clients whose issues forced them to revisit previously held notions about confidentiality. Few mental health professionals had faced situations as complex as HIV. Models of counseling and psychotherapy that were taught in graduate programs did not anticipate the ethical complexity of working with clients with HIV.

Here was a new disease, sexually transmitted and fatal, that at first did not even have a name. Knowledge about transmission of the virus was scant, and there was a great deal of public and professional alarm. In those early days, it was not uncommon for patients with HIV to languish in hospital rooms that staff members would not enter. Meals were left at the door, and beds often were not changed. The medical profession was caught off guard and was unable to find reliable treatments for the strange ailments that people with HIV experienced. Not since the early days of the drug explosion in the 1960s had the United States faced such a bewildering medical, psychological, and social dilemma. Beginning in the gay community, the initial and, to some extent, continuing challenge is to provide high-quality services to marginalized and oppressed patients whose access to resources is often limited.

The initial response of professional and community groups mirrored that seen in the 1960s. Traditional social services and medical agencies were reluctant to get involved for they did not know what to do, and they found themselves encountering a gay community about which little was actually known. Many medical and mental health professionals reacted to gay men through the negative stereotype that has existed for generations. Grass roots, peer-led organizations appeared in gay communities to try to lend assistance to a desperate population that could not find help elsewhere. The level of hysteria was fueled by media attention that reported the threat of HIV and accelerated a level of fear in the general population. Politicians and policy makers were confronted with a health crisis that demanded frank discussion of sexual practices and enormous sums of money. HIV challenged both community resources and individual humanity.

As clients began to appear for services in the early 1980s, about the only thing for certain in their treatment was that death would come quickly. In 1986, the average time between diagnosis and death was 8 months, and those months typically were filled with debilitating and strange illnesses; the client's reaction to physical symptoms and his struggle with stigmatization filled the largest portion of the counseling hour (Barret, 1989). Mental health practitioners found themselves confronting very complex treatment issues accompanied by complicated ethical issues. Duty to treat, duty to warn, dual relationships, and various end-of-life issues led many to avoid HIV-related psychotherapy. Practitioners were facing serious crises with little or no guidance from professional organizations, the research literature, or training programs. Ethics boards were similarly unprepared to respond for rarely had psychologists worked in such a cutting-edge environment where there was no standard of care.

Today, there is a better informed profession with a rapidly growing literature that gives insight into treatment issues. There are protocols that help the practitioner create a treatment plan. Still, although there is more familiarity with and agreement about treatment models, there are still very few resources for help with ethical issues. Practitioners no longer struggle over the duty to treat patients with HIV, and the entire level of service delivery has improved. However, mental health practitioners continue to grapple with the limits of confidentiality.

Consider the following two hypothetical client presentations:

> Miguel is a 36-year-old, heterosexually identified Hispanic client who went to a clinic after learning that his boyfriend, Carlos, had tested positive for HIV infection. Carlos and Miguel had been having unprotected sex for 2 years. Miguel does not want to be tested for HIV because he believes that he may have to tell his wife, Helena, about his secret life. Since learning that Carlos has HIV, Miguel says he has not had sex with Helena, who is 5 months pregnant with their second child. Miguel believes that there is little chance that Helena would be infected and spends most of his time in treatment talking about his confused feelings for Carlos. They continue to see each other twice per week for sex, but Miguel feels both angry and sad about the way their relationship has changed. Now he worries about having sex, and he knows that he needs to insist that they use protection. So far, that has not happened because Carlos does not like to use condoms.

A clinician treating Miguel is faced with a number of dilemmas. Is the number one priority to encourage him to be tested? Or must the mental health practitioner immediately insist that Helena be told? On the one hand, there is a very real danger that if pressure is applied to Miguel to tell his wife, he may terminate treatment and never return to the clinic. On the other hand, each day that Helena and her unborn child live without access to treatment for HIV may lead to increased risk. Determining a course of action in this situation is not easy. It is made more complex by the availability of medical treatments that have been proved to prolong life. Now that HIV is not necessarily fatal, early intervention is more important than ever; if their unborn child has HIV, then medical treatment may be able to eradicate the virus.

> Jason has lived with HIV disease for more than 10 years. His has been a courageous struggle, and he has become a role model for his community. He has lectured to community groups about the challenges of life with HIV disease, and his optimism has been an ever-present source of encouragement to many. During these years, he has been in and out of psychological treatment, building up a solid relationship with his counselor. Rejected by his family because of his homosexuality, Jason has surrounded himself with a loving support system of friends, medical and social support personnel, and

even people who know him only through his lectures. As others respond successfully to new medical advances, Jason deteriorates. He returns to his counselor as his physical and material resources dwindle. An assessment reveals no significant psychopathology or depression; Jason is functioning well within normal limits as he begins to discuss ending his own life with an overdose of pills. He is out of money and faces eviction from the apartment where he has lived for 6 years. His body is wasting rapidly, and his physician tells him that there is no longer anything that can be done. Death seems certain; the path to the end of his life is less clear in terms of time and suffering. Jason concludes that such pain is a waste and that he wants to end his life with as much dignity as possible. In the past 6 weeks, his health has deteriorated to the point that he now needs a full-time caregiver. On his good days, he functions pretty well, but when he is weak and despondent, he goes without eating and often is unable to get to the bathroom. He has told his closest friends that he wants to die and tried unsuccessfully to reconnect with his parents. His counselor struggles with understanding Jason's decision, respecting him for his strength, and confusion about breaking confidentiality to prevent his death.

Jason's counselor has a complex series of issues to resolve. Clearly there is a push to break confidentiality to prolong Jason's life. At the same time, there is a growing national debate about the right of terminally ill patients to be involved in deciding when and how to die (Rabkin, Remien, & Wilson, 1994). Still, the counselor who does not act to stop Jason from killing himself may face enormous ethical and legal sanctions. Determining what to do throws one into a social issue that is unresolved today. Stopping Jason may deprive him of a source of support that is essential as he heads toward death. Letting him execute his plan may leave the counselor with internal and external conflicts.

These two cases illustrate the most vexing aspects of confidentiality as applied to HIV-related psychotherapy. There is not a clear standard of care, there are few professionals who are willing to talk openly about how they manage such clients for fear of losing their licenses, and the advent of state laws regarding partner notification and assisted suicide intensifies the treatment dilemma. These two issues—deciding when to break confidentiality when a person with HIV continues to place others at risk through unsafe sex or needle sharing and deciding the proper role when faced with a terminally ill client who is wanting to end life—constitute the more intense debate about the limits of confidentiality.

THE CHALLENGE

In most ethical dilemmas, practitioners may hold out the hope that someone will have the answer that will lead to resolution, but in HIV-related psychotherapy, the course of action remains cloudy. As a standard of care is developed to suggest concrete ways of managing clients like Miguel and Jason, the situation will be much easier. For now, often the clinician must find his or her own way of deciding what to do. Looking at ethical codes, one finds the expected statements about protecting the client from harming him- or herself or others. Interpreting how this might be applied to Jason or Miguel does not really reveal a clear course of action. Those who contact ethics committees established by state boards find little help. Psychologists are often referred to the American Psychological Association's Office on AIDS as a potential consultant. Even when looking to the professional literature, the practitioner finds more complexity (Wood, Marks, & Dilley, 1990). Cohen (1995) reported that the tension between confidentiality and duty to warn remains and that even where disclosure may be mandated by law, there are instances when the counselor will choose not to breach confidentiality.

Consider the following questions that illustrate the complexity of this dilemma. How might one ethically manage an adolescent with HIV who does not want her legal guardian told of her infection but who speaks with her counselor about becoming sexually active with her boyfriend? What about the pregnant mother with HIV who refuses to let her physician know of her HIV status? Or how about the mother of an infant with HIV who does not want her child treated with medicines that may have harmful side effects? What is an appropriate course of action when faced with a client who has deteriorated to the point that he is unable to walk confidently yet continues to drive a car? What resources are available to the professional who is treating a woman with HIV whose income is gained through prostitution and who does not inform her sex partners that she is infected or insist that they use condoms? In each of these instances, the pressure to break confidentiality may be intense, yet there are often legal, ethical, and moral constraints that encourage the practitioner to remain silent.

Clinicians who work with adolescents with HIV face a special issue about confidentiality: disclosure to parents. Olson, Huszti, Mason, and Seibert (1989) explored the ethical issues surrounding disclosure of an adolescent's HIV diagnosis to parents. Gard (1990) examined the same topic but from a perspective of assisting adolescents with informing their parents. North (1990) presented a most comprehensive review of issues regarding testing and counseling adolescents without parental consent. This author argued for the availability of testing and counseling for adolescents and pointed out that the legal authority for this service exists in most states.

These dramas take place in all social institutions but especially in public health clinics and in institutional settings such as prisons and mental hospitals. By far, the most common issue is what to do with clients with HIV who continue to have unsafe sex (Pope & Vetter, 1992).

THE LIMITS OF CONFIDENTIALITY
WITH CLIENTS WITH HIV WHO PRACTICE UNSAFE SEX

The fundamental tension for the counselor who is faced with a client with HIV who reports continuing unsafe sex practices is to determine primary responsibility and the potential outcome of breaching confidentiality. Is the clinical obligation to work toward changing the client's behavior, or is it more fundamental that the public be protected? If confidentiality is breached, then what happens when the client discontinues treatment and continues his or her unsafe practices? Perhaps the mistrust that evolves leads others to avoid mental health treatment. The conflict between fidelity to the client and warning the public constitutes the dilemma. It is the most frequently reported tension for psychologists who work with clients with HIV (Cohen, 1990). Even though HIV disease is being seen as a chronic infection that may not lead to death, the intensity of these situations continues to be burdensome. In spite of the laws enacted in many states, the counselor must weigh various and perhaps conflicting options when deciding what to do.

In reviewing the literature related to confidentiality and HIV-related psychotherapy, the reader is advised to keep in mind the rapidly changing nature of HIV treatment. Issues that existed early in the epidemic have, in some cases, been ameliorated by changes in legislation and/or case law. In some states, practitioners are directed by state law to break confidentiality even when there is no identifiable victim. However, because the law varies from state to state, it is essential that mental health professionals know the situation in states where they practice. State laws also vary in determining the age at which adolescents own the right to privacy.

Now that more than 28 states have passed laws that require disclosure, one might think that the problem is solved, but an examination of case law reveals how the confusion continues. Even as late as 1998, there are few cases in which the law has addressed this question. Most practitioners fall back on other cases in which an individual or the public in general has been placed at risk. The most commonly cited reference on this issue is *Tarasoff v. Regents of the University of California* (1974, 1976), which held that the right to privacy ends where public peril begins. In instances in which harm seems imminent, exception to the restrictions of confidentiality are readily apparent.

As comforting as *Tarasoff v. Regents of the University of California* might be, subsequent court rulings have clarified the situations in which confidentiality may be broken. Breaching confidentiality is acceptable only when there is an identifiable victim and the stated intent of the client is to do harm (Burris, 1993). In Miguel's situation, it is obvious that he does not want to harm his wife, that she is not his victim. Does this mean that the counselor who informs Helena that Miguel has HIV has violated Miguel's right to privacy? Could such a disclosure result in a successful malpractice suit? Burris (in press) cautions about premature disclosure. In a court of law, can one prove that HIV was transmitted from Miguel to Helena? Perhaps she was infected elsewhere. Given the variable course of HIV infection, it could be possible that Helena has not yet been infected, in spite of exposure. The problem in applying the reasoning in *Tarasoff v. Regents of the University of California* to HIV is that virtually every state has on the books laws that limit access to knowledge of HIV infection, thereby preserving confidentiality; therefore, psychotherapists who place HIV information in a patient's records need to know the relevant state laws. Although many of these provisions are written in broad language, some are very detailed when it comes to notification of others about an individual's HIV status (Burris, 2000).

Knapp and VandeCreek (1989, 1990) discussed the failure of the courts to apply *Tarasoff v. Regents of the University of California* to cases involving HIV infection. They recommended that states adopt laws that would permit but not require warning potential victims. They, like others, argued that the potential benefits of keeping the client with HIV in treatment are enhanced by a relationship characterized by trust rather than distrust. Premature disclosure does little to help and may damage the client's reputation, deter others from seeking treatment, or cause those already in treatment to withhold information or even terminate treatment prematurely.

Perry (1989) argued that *Tarasoff v. Regents of the University of California* is not directly applicable because individuals with HIV do not have homicidal motives when they are sexually irresponsible. Also, the potential victims of this client have been exposed to a wide variety of media that clearly indicate the degree of risk in unprotected intercourse or needle sharing (Kain, 1988). Perry believed that applying *Tarasoff v. Regents of the University of California* to HIV-related psychotherapy merely creates an obstacle to building an effective therapeutic alliance and suggested that treatment is more likely to lead to behavior change.

Determining the degree of risk in breaking confidentiality in HIV-related situations involves assessing probabilities. Most people with HIV live in marginalized communities where the access to the kind of information about legal rights and the necessary funds to support a legal case are limited (Aiken & Musheno, 1994). Although there are some cases that have gone to court, their numbers are few and the decisions involved in them give little direction (Burris, 1993).

To determine the process used to resolve the limits of confidentiality, Totten, Lamb, and Reeder (1990) mailed to 1,000 practicing psychologists questionnaires with hypothetical scenarios dealing with varying degrees of danger and ability to identify the victim. Analysis of the 254 responses identified two groups. People who had not treated clients with HIV do use the *Tarasoff v. Regents of the University of California* guidelines but emphasize the degree of danger as more important than the ability to identify the victim when making a decision about breaching confidentiality. In their sample, clinicians who work routinely with clients with HIV were less likely to break confidentiality than the other group. Totten et al. (1990) reported that psychologists are more likely to break confidentiality when the client with HIV is either gay or a prostitute than when the client is bisexual or an intravenous drug user. This finding suggests the influence of prejudice in the decision-making process. Others (McGuire, Nieri, Abbot, Sheridan, & Fisher, 1995) echoed the influence of prejudice toward homosexuals and prostitutes in decisions about confidentiality.

The issue of confidentiality with clients with HIV is also complicated for prison populations. Skoler and Dargen (1990) identified the general helplessness of inmates with HIV in influencing administrative decisions about segregating, testing, and other restrictive measures for penal residents with HIV. Although the courts generally have been supportive of inmate claims of careless breaches of confidentiality, many penal institutions continue to create policies that treat inmates with HIV both unethically and illegally. Lurigio (1989), after surveying both probation and detention personnel, encouraged the creation of policy guidelines that delineate legal liability, confidentiality, mandatory testing, case contacts, and increased education of offenders and staff.

Confidentiality is especially complex when working with individuals in institutions. Hospitalized or incarcerated clients may be sexually active within the institution, placing other individuals at risk. Abramson (1990) interviewed 16 hospital social workers and found that secrecy about HIV infection was the main moral issue that caused distress for practitioners. Much of the secrecy surrounds topics such as the nature of the diagnosis, disclosure to other medical staff, disclosure to other patients, and the underlying issue of patient rights. Botello, Weinberger, and Gross (1990) outlined criteria that must be met when breaching confidentiality with individuals in institutions. First, they suggested that the client must be informed of his or her HIV seropositive status and of HIV-related safety practices. Second, the client must be diagnosed with a mental disorder that can significantly impair the client's ability to employ safe sex practices. These authors suggested that confidentiality be breached only when these conditions are met. Haimowitz (1989), in reviewing issues related to the treatment of individuals with mental illness, suggested that HIV testing and disclosure without informed consent should be strictly limited and conducted only when clinically necessary.

Perhaps the most extensive discussion of ethical issues in working with clients with HIV was offered by Appelbaum and Appelbaum (1990). Although they addressed the topic from the perspective of medically based psychiatric treatment, they examined the conflict between confidentiality and the protection of others, the clash between ethical principles and professional guidelines, the lack of statutory action, and the management of both in- and outpatients who have HIV. Zonana (1989) reviewed similar issues and pointed out that it is the prevalence of stigmatization and discrimination directed toward people with HIV that makes the decision about breaking confidentiality so complex.

Adler and Beckett (1989) presented a brief but interesting discussion of society's rights versus patients' rights and concluded by encouraging professional organizations to identify more specific guidelines for breaking confidentiality in HIV cases. They, along with others (Appelbaum & Appelbaum, 1990; Erickson, 1993; Gray & Harding, 1988), argued that the rights of the endangered override the rights of the client because of the fatal nature of HIV. Although this disease now is seen more as a chronic infection, it is important to recognize that the rights of the endangered still may justify breaching confidentiality. Winiarski (1991) encouraged psychotherapists to take a prevention stance that encourages keeping the client in treatment with the hope that behavior can be changed. Winiarski's bottom line is that confidentiality should be breached only when attempts at behavior change clearly have failed. Even then, the client must be informed that the breach is going to occur. The clinician is left to ponder these issues to come to some resolution that contains a course of action that can be defended professionally, ethically, and legally.

Knapp and VandeCreek (1993) suggested that when hospitalizing a client with HIV who is having unsafe sex, it is best to hospitalize on the basis of severe mental disorder rather than disclose the client's HIV status. They also suggested that the clinician speak openly to the client about concerns for endangered third parties and that confidentiality should be breached with the client's knowledge and in the client's presence. They concluded by warning practitioners who do breach confidentiality in HIV-related cases that they are not protected by law and that they must be prepared to *prove* that the client *intends* to infect others. Lamb, Clark, Drumheller, Frizzell, and Surrey (1989) echoed these concerns and encouraged psychologists to get training in working with individuals with HIV.

Cohen developed a set of guidelines that he believes help clinicians to decide what to do. Among his ethical rules are five statements:

1. There is medical evidence based on state-of-the-art testing criteria indicating that the client is HIV positive.
2. The third party is engaging in a relationship with the client such as unprotected sexual intercourse, which, according to current medical standards, places the third party at high risk of contracting HIV from the client.
3. The third party can be identified and contacted by the counselor without the intervention of law enforcement.
4. The client has refused to disclose to the third party and is not likely to do so in the near future, nor is anyone other than the counselor likely to do so.
5. As far as the clinician is aware, the third party is not him- or herself engaging in risky sexual behavior, such as promiscuous sex without the use of a condom. (1995, p. 250)

Cohen's procedure includes counselor options such as encouraging the client to disclose, disclosing only to the third party through a person-to-person contact, and offering counseling to the third party or making an appropriate referral.

Gray and Harding (1988) encouraged the practitioner to break confidentiality when a client with HIV is endangering the health of others by having unprotected intercourse, after first informing the client of the intent to break confidentiality and then informing known partners. In cases of anonymous partners, they suggested contacting the state or local health department official and informing appropriate civil and professional authorities. Responding to this article, Kain (1988) suggested caution when working with gay men. First, the practitioner is advised not to assume that gay equals seropositive status, and, second, he pointed out that few clients with HIV are likely to reveal either sex practices or health status when advised that such disclosures could lead to breaking confidentiality. He encouraged practitioners to investigate the reasons for not disclosing health status to sex partners. If breaching confidentiality is necessary, then the clinician is encouraged to offer treatment to those who are informed that they have been exposed to HIV infection.

Guidelines such as these may be the future when it comes to breaking confidentiality with a sexually irresponsible client with HIV. The fact remains that although more than 28 states have enacted legislation that demands disclosure to people who are at risk of HIV infection, there still are going to be situations in which the clinician will have to decide what to do. Each client must be seen as an individual, and mental health practitioners who are working with people with HIV disease will continue to struggle until the standard of care becomes more well defined.

RATIONAL SUICIDE

Nearly absent in the literature are articles that address confidentiality issues when the client is considering suicide. Perhaps this topic is not covered because society as a whole is having a difficult time determining both the legal and ethical rights of the terminally ill person who chooses suicide over treatment. There is neither an emerging consensus nor clear guidelines to help the practitioner decide what action to take. The norm continues to be that preventing suicide is the preeminent standard of care (Werth, 1992). Most people who provide psychological services to people with HIV disease report that thoughts and plans of suicide are commonplace (Cote, Biggar, & Dannenberg, 1992; Kalichman & Sikkeman, 1994).

Werth and Liddle (1994), in the report of their survey of the members of the American Psychological Association's division of psychotherapy, found that psychologists are less negative toward suicide when the clients are terminally ill. Eighty percent of their respondents answered affirmatively to their question, "Do you believe in the idea of rational suicide?"

Rabkin et al. (1994) explored the issue of physician-assisted suicide. According to their studies, HIV patients may turn to their physicians for help in ending their lives. In fact, some physicians are providing that assistance, through either withholding care or the use of pain medicines, such as morphine. Even professional organizations such as the American Psychological Association have established committees to examine end-of-life issues, and the National Association of Social Workers (1993) has a policy statement about end-of-life issues that does not mandate breaching confidentiality. More than 17 states have laws forbidding assisted suicide (Young, 1992). As of 1999, Oregon remains the only state that has enacted legislation that allows physician-assisted suicide (Colburn, 1994). Still, the American Psychological Association (1997) warned that thoughts of suicide may, in fact, be the effects of a treatable depression. It is also noteworthy that such thoughts of suicide may be related to HIV's attack on the central nervous system (Rogers & Britten, 1994).

In the midst of such ambiguity and social uneasiness with rational suicide, Werth (1995) offered a framework of "check points" to assist clinicians in deciding whether to break confidentiality with terminally ill clients who are considering suicide. Building on Siegel's (1986) model, Werth posited the following criteria for clinicians to consider:

1. The client can make a realistic assessment of the situation.
2. The client's mental processes are unimpaired by psychological illness or emotional distress.
3. The motivation of the client is understandable to a majority of uninvolved community members.
4. The decision has been contemplated and discussed over a period of time.
5. When it is possible, significant others should actively participate in the decision-making process.

Although using these criteria may not protect clinicians from legal action, the five factors may become the basis for creating a standard of care for end-of-life decisions.

Fortunately, given the improved medical treatment of people with HIV disease, assisted suicide is no longer as common an issue. However, the long-term impact of contemporary treatments is not clear, and it is possible that HIV infection may once again be seen as terminal. Mental health practitioners are encouraged to question Werth's (1995) criteria because such end-of-life decisions are likely to be contaminated by psychological and emotional distress and may be transitory. Still, there certainly are instances, such as that posed by Jason, in which the mental health practitioner will face and have to resolve this issue. Once again, this clinician will be on the cutting edge of the profession and may become a part of creating a new standard of care.

CONCLUSION

In most areas of mental health, decisions about breaking confidentiality benefit from precedence, the availability of informed colleagues for consultation, a body of literature that analyzes the various issues, legal cases that provide information about the level of risk, and experienced ethical board members. These resources continue to be in short supply for professionals who provide direct service to people with HIV. Practitioners who work with clients with HIV find themselves in a constantly changing environment in which the parameters of confidentiality likewise continue to shift. As experience is gained and as medical treatments become more predictable, it is hoped that the standard of care as it relates to the principle of confidentiality will become, in fact, more standard. Until that time comes, professionals must exercise extreme caution when faced with situations that challenge the limits of confidentiality.

REFERENCES

Abramson, M. (1990). Keeping secrets: Social workers and AIDS. *Social Work, 35*(2), 169–173.

Adler, G., & Beckett, A. (1989). Psychotherapy of the patient with an HIV infection: Some ethical and therapeutic dilemmas. *Psychometrics, 33*(2), 203–208.

Aiken, J., & Musheno, M. (1994). Why have-nots win in HIV-litigation areas: Socio-legal dynamics of extreme cases. *Law and Policy, 16*, 267–297.

American Psychological Association. (1997). *Terminal illness and hastened death requests: The important role of the mental health professional.* Washington, DC: Author.

Appelbaum, K., & Appelbaum, P. (1990). The HIV antibody–positive patient. In J. Beck (Ed.), *Confidentiality versus the duty to protect: Foreseeable harm in the practice of psychiatry* (pp. 121–140). Washington, DC: American Psychiatric Press.

Barret, R. (1989). Counseling gay men with AIDS: Human dimensions. *Journal of Counseling and Development, 67*(10), 573–575.

Botello, T., Weinberger, L., & Gross, B. (1990). A proposed exception to the AIDS confidentiality laws for psychiatric patients. *Journal of Forensic Sciences, 35*(3), 653–661.

Burris, S. (1993). Testing, disclosure, and the right to privacy. In S. Burris & J.L. Miller (Eds.), *AIDS law today* (pp. 3–17). New Haven, CT: Yale University Press.

Burris, S. (2000). Clinical decision-making in the shadow of the law. In J. Anderson & R. Barret (Eds.), *Ethical issues in HIV-related therapy.* Washington, DC: American Psychological Association.

Cohen, E. (1990). Confidentiality, counseling, and clients who have AIDS: Ethical foundations of a model rule. *Journal of Counseling and Development, 68*(3), 282–286.

Cohen, E. (1995). Ethical standards counseling sexually active clients with HIV. In W. Odets & M. Shernoff (Eds.), *The second decade of AIDS: A mental health practitioner handbook* (pp. 233–254). New York: Hatherleigh Press.

Colburn, D. (1994, November 15). Assisted suicide bill passes. *The Washington Post,* p. Z9.

Cote, T.R., Biggar, R.J., & Dannenberg, A.L. (1992). Risk of suicide among patients with AIDS: A national assessment. *Journal of the American Medical Association, 268,* 2066–2068.

Erickson, S.H. (1993). Ethics and confidentiality in AIDS counseling: A professional dilemma. *Journal of Mental Health Counseling, 15*(2), 118–131.

Gard, L. (1990). Patient disclosure of human immunodeficiency virus (HIV) status to parents: Clinical considerations. *Professional Psychology: Research and Practice, 21*(4), 252–256.

Gray, L.A., & Harding, A.K. (1988). Confidentiality limits with clients who have the AIDS virus. *Journal of Counseling and Development, 66*(5), 219–223.

Haimowitz, S. (1989). HIV and the mentally ill: An approach to the legal issues. *Hospital and Community Psychiatry, 40*(7), 732–736.

Kain, C.D. (1988). To breach or not to breach? A response to Gray and Harding. *Journal of Counseling and Development, 66*(5), 224–225.

Kalichman, S.C., & Sikkeman, K.J. (1994). Psychological sequelae of HIV infection and AIDS: Review of empirical findings. *Clinical Psychological Review, 14*(7), 611–632.

Knapp, S., & VandeCreek, L. (1989). What psychologists need to know about AIDS. *Journal of Training and Practice in Professional Psychology, 3*(2), 3–16.

Knapp, S., & VandeCreek, L. (1990). Application of the duty to protect to HIV-positive clients. *Professional Psychology: Research and Practice, 21*(3), 161–166.

Knapp, S., & VandeCreek, L. (1993). Legal and ethical issues in billing patients and collecting fees. *Psychotherapy, 30*(1), 25–31.

Lamb, D., Clark, C., Drumheller, P., Frizzell, K., & Surrey, L. (1989). Applying Tarasoff to AIDS-related psychotherapy issues. *Professional Psychology: Research and Practice, 20*(1), 37–43.

Lurigio, A.J. (1989). Practitioners' views on AIDS and probation and detention. *Federal Probation, 53*(4), 16–24.

McGuire, J., Nieri, D., Abbot, D., Sheridan, K., & Fisher, R. (1995). Do Tarasoff principles apply in AIDS-related psychotherapy? Ethical decision making and the role of therapist homophobia and perceived client dangerousness. *Professional Psychology: Research and Practice, 26*(6), 608–611.

National Association of Social Workers. (1993). *Social work speaks: NASW policy statements.* Washington, DC: Author.

North, R. (1990). Legal authority for HIV testing of adolescents. *Journal of Adolescent Health Care, 11*(2), 176–187.

Olson, R., Huszti, H., Mason, P., & Seibert, J. (1989). Pediatric AIDS/HIV infection: An emerging challenge to pediatric psychology. *Journal of Pediatric Psychology, 14*(1), 1–21.

Perry, S. (1989). AIDS and confidentiality: Legal concept and its application in psychotherapy [Comment]. *American Journal of Psychotherapy, 43*(3), 462.

Pope, K.S., & Vetter, V.A. (1992). Ethical dilemmas encountered by members of the American Psychological Association: A national survey. *American Psychologist, 47*, 397–411.

Rabkin, J., Remien, R., & Wilson, C. (1994). *Good doctors, good patients: Partners in HIV treatment.* New York: NCM Publishers.

Rogers, J.R., & Britten, P.J. (1994). AIDS and rational suicide: A counseling psychology perspective or a slide on a slippery slope. *The Counseling Psychologist, 22*(1), 171–178.

Siegel, K. (1986). Psychosocial aspects of rational suicide. *American Journal of Psychotherapy, 40*, 405–418.

Skoler, D., & Dargen, R. (1990). AIDS in prisons: Administrator policies, inmate protests, and reactions from the federal bench. *Federal Probation, 54*(2), 27–32.

Tarasoff v. Regents of the University of California, 529 P.2d 553 (Cal. 1974); 551 P.2d 334, 331 (Cal. 1976).

Totten, G., Lamb, D., & Reeder, G. (1990). "Tarasoff" and confidentiality in AIDS-related psychotherapy. *Professional Psychology: Research and Practice, 21*(3), 155–160.

Werth, J.L., Jr. (1992). Rational suicide and AIDS: Considerations for the psychotherapist. *The Counseling Psychologist, 20*(4), 645–659.

Werth, J.L., Jr. (1995). Rational suicide reconsidered: AIDS as an impetus for change. *Death Studies, 19*(1), 65–80.

Werth, J.L., Jr., & Liddle, B.J. (1994). Psychotherapist's attitude towards suicide. *Psychotherapy: Theory, Research and Practice, 31*(3), 440–448.

Winiarski, M. (1991). *AIDS-related psychotherapy.* New York: Pergamon.

Wood, G.J., Marks, R., & Dilley, J.W. (1990). *AIDS law for mental health professionals: A handbook for judicious practice.* San Francisco: AIDS Health Project.

Young, H.H. (1992). Assisted suicide and physician liability. *The Review of Litigation, 11*, 623–656.

Zonana, H. (1989). The duty to protect: Confidentiality and HIV. In J. Dilley, C. Pies, & M. Helquist (Eds.), *Face to face: A guide to AIDS counseling* (pp. 219–229). Berkeley, CA: Celestial Arts.

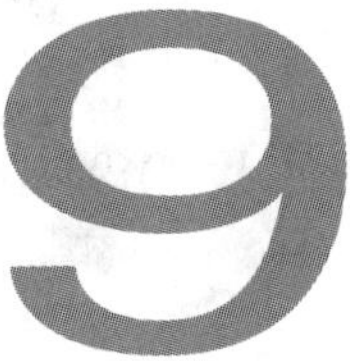

Confidentiality of Alcohol
and Other Drug Patient Records

Paul N. Samuels

On August 14, 1998, in Fairfax County, Virginia, police officers entered a drug treatment program, turning away patients who had been waiting for care for hours and seizing photographs, treatment schedules, and other patient information. The police were investigating the theft of a ring from a jewelry store by an unknown man who was seen stealing a car and driving off. According to the *Washington Post,* "several office buildings are closer than the . . . Treatment Clinic to the spot where the car was taken, and police did not give any other reason to suspect anyone connected with the clinic" (Masters, 1998, p. C1).

The lack of any evidence linking anyone at the treatment program with the crime probably makes the search warrant that the police had obtained from a magistrate invalid under the Fourth Amendment to the U.S. Constitution, which prohibits unreasonable searches and seizures. Just as egregious, the police failed to obtain the authorizing court order required by the federal statute and regulations protecting alcohol and other drug abuse patient records (42 U.S.C. § 290dd-2 and 42 C.F.R. "Confidentiality of Records" Part 2). The original version of this law was passed in 1972 to provide stringent federal privacy protections for people entering alcohol and other drug treatment and prevention programs. Explaining the need for this nationally applicable law, its congressional sponsors stressed that:

> The strictest adherence to the provisions of this [law] is absolutely es-
> sential to the success of all drug abuse . . . programs. Every patient and
> former patient must be assured that his right to privacy will be pro-
> tected. Without that assurance, fear of public disclosure of drug abuse
> or of records that will attach for life will discourage thousands from
> seeking the treatment they must have if this tragic national problem is
> to be overcome. ("Confidentiality of Records" H.R. Rep. No. 920)

Recognizing their errors, the Fairfax County law enforcement authorities returned the illegally seized records to the treatment program. The damage caused to the traumatized patients is harder to redress.

Twenty-six years earlier and hundreds of miles to the north, the New York County (Manhattan) District Attorney's Office served a subpoena on Dr. Robert Newman, then Director of the New York City Methadone Maintenance Treatment Program, requiring him to produce photographs of "Negro males between the ages of 21 and 35" who were patients in one of his programs. Motivated by what New York State's highest court later agreed was "the highest ethical canons of the medical profession in respect of confidentiality relations with a patient," Dr. Newman was held in contempt of court and sentenced to 30 days in jail when he refused to comply with the subpoena. He appealed, and both the subpoena and the contempt citation were thrown out.

Although this case was decided under an earlier statute that provided absolute confidentiality, the New York court expressed its agreement with the statement in the just-enacted federal confidentiality regulations that "if society is to make significant progress in the struggle against drug abuse, 'the directors of drug abuse treatment programs' must be able 'to assure patients and prospective patients of anonymity'" (*People v. Newman*, 1973).

The Fairfax County incident demonstrates just how prescient were the drafters of the federal confidentiality law and regulations (hereinafter referred to collectively as "the federal confidentiality rules") and the judges of the New York Court of Appeals, for stigma and prejudice continue to haunt the way many people—even within the justice system—view people who experience alcohol and other drug dependence. Consider what the Fairfax County detective who obtained the tainted warrant to search the drug treatment program stated in his affidavit to the magistrate explaining why he sought that warrant: "It is common for people who have addictions of various narcotics . . . to engage in these kinds of criminal activities to support [their] drug addictions" (Masters, 1998, p. C1). That patients in a treatment program are confronting their addiction and perhaps should not automatically be considered criminals seems to have escaped the detective's attention completely.

Such biased attitudes did not escape the attention of the drafters of the federal confidentiality rules, fortunately for those with or at risk for alcohol and other drug problems and for the United States as a whole. If the federal confidentiality rules did not exist—and law enforcement officials and others were able to obtain patient records as readily as they can obtain other health care records—many, perhaps even most, people in need of alcohol and other drug treatment and prevention services would be afraid to come forward to obtain those services. That is why Congress enacted the only *federal* law in the area of confidentiality. At least for now, the privacy of all other health care services provided by non-federal government agencies is governed by state and local laws, not federal.

As noted previously, the federal confidentiality rules were first enacted in the early 1970s. Although violation of the federal confidentiality rules carries criminal penalties, the requirements largely are self-enforced. Those who maintain or seek alcohol or other drug patient records have the obligation to disclose or redisclose patient information only as permitted by the federal rules. As a result, familiarity with the confidentiality regulations is essential for anyone directly or indirectly involved with alcohol or other drug abuse prevention or treatment, including mental health, public health, criminal justice, welfare, child welfare, and many other professionals and agencies.

PATIENT NOTICE OF CONFIDENTIALITY RULES AND REGULATIONS

The federal confidentiality rules require programs to notify patients of the existence of the law and regulations and to give them a written summary. The notice and summary should be provided at admission or "as soon thereafter as the patient is capable of rational communication" (42 C.F.R. "Confidentiality of Records" 2.22 Title 42 § 2.22[a]).

The regulations list five items that must be included in the written summary and notice:

> 1) A description of the few circumstances in which disclosures can be made without consent, 2) a statement that violation of the regulations is a reportable crime, 3) a warning that information can be released if the patient commits or threatens a crime on program premises or against program personnel, 4) a notice that the program must report suspected child abuse or neglect, and 5) a citation to the law and regulations. (Id. § 2.22[b])

DEFINITIONS AND BASIC REQUIREMENTS OF DISCLOSURE

Except under specified conditions, the federal confidentiality rules prohibit the disclosure of records or other information concerning any patient in a federally assisted alcohol or other drug abuse program (42 C.F.R. "Confidentiality of Records" 2.22 Title 42 §§ 2.12, 2.13[a]). This prohibition on unauthorized disclosure applies regardless of whether the person seeking information already has the information, has other means of obtaining it, enjoys official status, has obtained a subpoena or warrant, or is authorized by state law (Id. §§ 2.13[b], 2.20). Any state provision that would permit or require a disclosure that is prohibited by the federal rules is invalid. However, the federal rules permit states to require greater confidentiality than the federal regulations (Id. § 2.20).

Patients whose records are protected by the federal confidentiality rules include any person who has applied for, participated in, or received an interview, counseling, or any other service from a federally assisted alcohol or other drug abuse program. Applicants are included, regardless of whether they are admitted to treatment. Former patients and deceased patients are also protected (Id. §§ 2.11, 2.15[b]).

The federal rules even protect the confidentiality of records gathered from the evaluation of eligibility for treatment or provision of that treatment for someone arrested on a criminal charge. In *Jeanette "A" v. Condon* (1989), the court refused to allow a positive urinalysis test for cocaine to be used by the police department in a proceeding to discharge a police officer. The court found that the urinalysis test was covered by the federal confidentiality law because it was administered as part of a treatment regimen, pointing out that "Congress sought to protect the privacy of people so that they would enroll in treatment programs" (Id. at 207).

The confidentiality rules do *not* apply to urine or blood tests for alcohol or other drugs if those tests are *not* administered during the course of providing treatment. For example, in *State v. Friedman* (1998), the Tennessee Court of Criminal Appeals allowed the results of blood alcohol tests conducted by a hospital emergency room on a man arrested for driving under the influence to be introduced at his trial. The court based its ruling on the fact that the defendant "failed to show that the records . . . pertain to activities related to treatment and prevention of substance abuse" (Id. at 5).

If a program receives a request for a disclosure of an individual's records that is not permitted by the regulations, then it must refuse to make the disclosure and must be sure to do so in a way that does not reveal that the individual has ever been diagnosed or treated for alcohol or other drug abuse. An appropriate response is, "Federal law prohibits me from disclosing that information."

The program is allowed to give inquiring parties copies of the regulations and explain that they restrict disclosure of alcohol and other drug abuse patient records, as long as the program does not affirmatively identify a particular individual as a patient whose records are confidential. However, if the individual who is the subject of the inquiry is not and never has been a patient, the program can reveal that fact (42 C.F.R. "Confidentiality of Records" 2.22 Title 42 § 2.13[c][2]).

Program is defined by the regulations to include any person or organization that, in whole or in part, provides alcohol or other drug abuse diagnosis, treatment, or referral for treatment *and* receives "federal assistance" (including federal funding and tax-exempt status). Thus, a federally assisted community mental health center that provides alcohol or other drug services to some or all of its patients would have to follow the federal confidentiality rules when handling or disclosing patient information concerning those patients.

Patient records maintained by a hospital or medical center are not covered under the regulations unless the patient receives treatment (or diagnosis or referral for treatment) from 1) a specialized alcohol or other drug abuse unit of the hospital or medical center or 2) medical personnel or other staff whose primary function is to provide services for alcohol or other drug abuse. Thus, patients in the general population or emergency room of a hospital or medical center, even if diagnosed as having an alcohol or other drug abuse problem, frequently will not be protected (Id. § 2.11).

The federal confidentiality rules strictly limit the information that can be disclosed by programs covered under the rules. Any communication of information about an identified patient or of information that would identify someone as a patient or as an alcohol or other drug abuser, including verification of information that is already known by the person making the inquiry, is covered and can be disclosed only as authorized by the rules (Id. §§ 2.11, 2.12[a][1][I]).

Implicit, as well as explicit, disclosures are prohibited (Id. § 2.13[c]). For example, one may not disclose that a particular individual is attending a program that is publicly identified as a place where only alcohol or other drug abuse services are provided, unless the individual consents in accordance with the regulations or unless the disclosure is otherwise authorized. Accordingly, all requests for unauthorized disclosures about patients should be met with a noncommittal response (e.g., "federal law prohibits the release of that information").

Records that are protected from unauthorized disclosure include any information acquired about a patient, whether it is in writing or recorded in some other form or not, including the patient's identity, address, medical or treatment information, and all communications made by him or her to program staff (Id. § 2.11). This means that the memories and impressions of program staff are considered "records" that are protected by the regulations even if they are never recorded in any form.

To protect the privacy of patients and encourage them to enter therapy without fear of retribution or embarrassment, *all* information gathered by an alcohol or other drug treatment program is protected and can be disclosed only as authorized by the federal confidentiality rules. To illustrate, in *In re Commissioner of Social Services v. David S.* (1982), the New York City Commissioner of Social Services brought a paternity proceeding against David S. on behalf of Guiliana S. To impeach her credibility in the paternity suit by showing prior pregnancies and a history of promiscuity, David sought to subpoena records regarding Guiliana, the mother, from a youth counseling center that provided her with treatment for alcohol and other drug abuse. The New York Court of Appeals upheld the treatment program's refusal to disclose the records, stating that preserving the confidentiality of all information gathered while providing alcohol and other drug treatment services was essential to "further the objective of the federal statute addressing drug and alcohol abuse treatment . . . by not chilling the willingness or discouraging the readiness of individuals to come to facilities operated under the statute."

Everyone who has access to patients' records is obligated to know and follow the federal confidentiality rules—treatment program personnel, researchers, auditors, and others. The rules apply to them, regardless of whether they are compensated for their activity, and continue to apply to them after they have terminated their employment or relationship with the program.

RULES FOR MAKING DISCLOSURES

The federal confidentiality rules set out a number of conditions permitting limited disclosures upon patient consent and a few circumstances in which disclosures may be made regardless of whether the patient consents. In general, they fall into nine categories: written consent; court order; child abuse and neglect reporting; internal communications; no patient-identifying information; medical emergency; crime at program or against program personnel; research, audit, or evaluation; and Qualified Service Organization Agreement. Each condition has its own peculiar requirements and limitations, all of practical significance.

The rules permitting disclosure present relatively complicated questions, and some are not easily subject to generalized answers. One practical step toward minimizing confidentiality problems is to inform program personnel that, other than in such routine situations as when the patient signs a valid consent form, only the program director or some designated individual versed in the confidentiality regulations may authorize disclosures. Even then, certain situations, particularly those involving court orders, may require the advice of counsel.

To determine whether a particular request for information about a patient falls within one of the exceptions to the general prohibition on disclosure, one should ask the following questions:

1. Has the patient executed a proper consent form for the proposed communication?
2. Is the proposed communication to be made to other staff of the program or to an entity with direct administrative control over the program?
3. Can the proposed communication be made without revealing that the person whom the disclosure concerns is or was a patient or an alcohol or other drug abuser?
4. Is the proposed communication needed to respond to a medical emergency?
5. Is the proposed communication authorized by a valid court order?
6. Does the proposed communication concern a crime or a threatened crime on the premises of the program or against program personnel?
7. Is the proposed communication for purposes of research or part of an audit or an evaluation of a program's activities?
8. Does the proposed communication involve the reporting of child abuse or neglect?
9. Will the proposed communication be made pursuant to a Qualified Service Organization Agreement?

If the answer to all of these questions is no, then the proposed communication probably *cannot* be made. If, however, the answer to one of the questions is yes, then the situation may permit a disclosure if certain conditions are met and certain procedures are followed. An examination of each of these nine exceptions follows.

Written Consent

The most common method of authorizing disclosure under the federal confidentiality rules is via a written consent form signed by the patient. Verbal consents are not permitted. In fact, even a simply worded "general release form" of the type used by most health care practitioners and insurance companies is *not* valid under the federal rules for authorizing disclosure of alcohol and other drug patient records. Instead, the federal rules require a significantly more detailed consent form that enables the patient to understand fully what is to be disclosed, to whom, and why. The requirement of a substantially more detailed consent form is perhaps the most significant departure in the federal rules for alcohol and other drug patient records from the confidentiality requirements for other forms of health care records, whether general practice, hospital, mental health, or other specialty.

Proper Format for Consent to Release Information   A proper consent form must contain *each* of the items specified in 42 C.F.R. 2.22 Title 42 § 2.31:

1. The name or general designation of the program(s) making the disclosure
2. The name of the individual or organization that will receive the disclosure
3. The name of the patient who is the subject of the disclosure
4. The purpose or need for the disclosure
5. How much and what kind of information will be disclosed
6. A statement that the patient may revoke the consent at any time, except to the extent that the program has already acted in reliance on it
7. The date, event, or condition on which the consent expires if not previously revoked
8. The signature of the patient (and/or other authorized person)
9. The date on which the consent is signed

As discussed previously, a general medical release form or any other consent form that does not contain all of the listed elements is not acceptable.

Understanding the Consent Requirements   Several of the items that must be included in a consent form merit further explanation:

1) the purpose of the disclosure and 2) how much and what kind of information will be disclosed. These two items are closely related. All disclosures, especially those made pursuant to a consent form, must be limited to information that is necessary to accomplish the need or purpose for the disclosure (42 C.F.R. "Confidentiality of Records" 2.22 Title 42 § 2.13[a]). It would be improper to disclose everything in a patient's file if the recipient of the information needs only one specific piece of information.

In completing a consent form, the person who is requesting the information must determine first the purpose or need for the communication of information. Once this has been identified, it is easier to determine how much and what kind of information will be disclosed, tailoring it to what is essential to accomplish the need or purpose that has been identified.

For example, if a patient needs to have the fact that he or she is in treatment verified in order to continue to receive government benefits, then the purpose of the disclosure would be "verification of current treatment status." The disclosure would then be limited to a statement that "John Smith (the patient) is in treatment at XYZ program as of September 10, 1999."

The consent form indicates that the patient may revoke consent at any time. Revocation need not be in writing. If a program has already made a disclosure prior to the revocation, then the program has acted in reliance on the consent and is not required to try to retrieve the information that it has already disclosed.

The regulations state that "acting in reliance" includes providing services in reliance on a consent form permitting disclosures to a third-party payer (Id. § 2.31[a][8]). Thus, a program can bill the third-party payer for past services to the patient even after consent has been revoked. However, a program that continues to provide services after a patient has revoked a consent authorizing disclosure to a third-party payer does so at its own financial peril.

The form must also contain a date, event, or condition on which it will expire if not previously revoked. A consent must last "no longer than reasonably necessary to serve the purpose for which it is given" (Id. § 2.31[a][9]). The consent form does not need to contain a specific expiration date but may instead specify an event or a condition, such as "until the patient is no longer eligible for insurance reimbursement."

Although the requirement of the patient's signature is easily fulfilled in most cases, there can be complications when the patient is a minor or when the patient is incompetent or deceased. Disclosures of records concerning minor patients require the written consent of the minor. The confidentiality regulations leave entirely to state laws the issue of who is a minor and whether a minor can obtain alcohol or other drug abuse treatment without the consent of a parent or other legal guardian. However, the regulations state that parental consent for disclosure to a third party (in addition to the minor's consent, not instead of it) is required only if the program is required by state law to obtain parental permission before providing treatment to the minor (Id. § 2.14).

The minor's written consent is usually required even when the disclosure is to be made to the minor's parents. Thus, in most circumstances, by withholding consent, a minor can prevent disclosure of information to a parent or other legal guardian about alcohol or other drug services that he or she received.

In the case of a patient who has been adjudicated incompetent to manage his or her affairs, consent to disclosures of alcohol or other drug abuse treatment records may be made by the individual's guardian or other person authorized by the state to act on his or her behalf. In such a situation, the patient's consent is not required (Id. § 2.15[a][1]).

If the patient has not been adjudicated incompetent but the program director determines that his or her medical condition prevents "knowing or effective action on his or her own behalf," then the program director may authorize disclosures without patient consent for the sole purpose of obtaining payment for services from a third-party payer—but for no other purpose without a court adjudication (Id. § 2.15[a][2]).

One of the most striking examples of the grave concern exhibited throughout the federal confidentiality rules that failure to provide assurances of confidentiality would deter people from entering addiction treatment is that even records of deceased patients remain confidential. As the United States Court of Appeals for the First Circuit stated in *Whyte v. Connecticut Mutual Life Insurance Co.* (1987), when ruling that life insurance beneficiaries could not obtain the treatment records of a deceased patient to prove his death was accidental rather than a suicide because the records are confidential even after the patient's death,

> While it is true that disclosure cannot harm [the deceased patient], it can harm his family and his reputation. In addition, the fear of post mortem disclosure may dissuade others who need treatment from seeking help or may prevent them from communicating with program personnel with the candor necessary for effective treatment. (Id. at p. 1010 n.13)

Consent to the disclosure of records of deceased patients may be made by the executor, administrator, or other personal representative appointed by will or by a court to manage the deceased patient's estate. If no personal representative has been appointed, then the patient's spouse or, if none, any responsible family member may give the required consent (42 C.F.R. "Confidentiality of Records" 2.22 Title 42 § 2.15[b][2]). Even without consent, a program may make limited disclosures about deceased patients when required by federal or state laws providing for the collection of vital statistics or an inquiry into the cause of death (Id. § 2.15[b][1]).

Written Prohibition on Redisclosure   Once a consent form has been properly completed, there remains one last formal requirement. Any disclosure made with written patient consent must be accompanied by a written statement that the information disclosed is protected by federal law and that the recipient cannot make any further disclosure of it unless permitted by the regulations (42 C.F.R. "Confidentiality of Records" 2.22 Title 42 § 2.32). This statement, not the consent form itself, should be delivered and explained to the recipient at the time of disclosure.

The prohibition on rediTsclosure is clear and strict. Those who receive the notice are prohibited from rereleasing information except as permitted by the regulations. (Of course, a patient may sign a consent form authorizing such a redisclosure.) The regulations prohibit redisclosure by a third-party payer or by an entity that has direct administrative control over a program even if it has not received the written notice (Id. § 2.12[d][2]). However, programs are still required to attach the notice prohibiting redisclosure to *all* disclosures made with patient consent, regardless of who is receiving the information.

Use of Consent Forms   The fact that a patient has signed a proper consent form authorizing the release of information does not *force* a program to make the proposed disclosure, unless the program has also received a subpoena or court order (42 C.F.R. 2.22 Title 42 §§ 2.3[b]; 2.61[a][b]). The program's only obligation is to refuse to honor a consent that is expired, deficient, or known to be revoked, false, or invalid (Id. § 2.31[c]).

In most cases, the decision to make a disclosure pursuant to a consent form is within the discretion of the program. It is important to note, however, that patients cannot properly consent to release of information for the purpose of criminal investigation or prosecution. Subsection c of the federal confidentiality statute ("Confidentiality of Records" 42 U.S.C. § 290dd-2[c] and § 2.12[d][1]) of the regulations prohibit use of information protected by the regulations in any criminal investigation or prosecution of a patient unless the court issues an authorizing order under § 2.65, regardless of consent. In general, it is best to follow this rule: Disclose only what is necessary, for only as long as is necessary, in light of the purpose of the communication.

The regulations allow a program to release any information about a patient who consents, even if there are potentially adverse consequences. For example, a program may, with patient consent, provide periodic progress reports to an employer, even if the reports mention continued substance abuse, refusal to cooperate with the program, or other deleterious information. However, given the stigma that some employers and others attach to alcohol and other drug abuse treatment, programs may wish to withhold disclosures from employers or others who they know will take adverse action against anyone with an alcohol or other drug abuse problem or history, at least until the program carefully considers the individual circumstances.

Special Rules for Criminal Justice System Referrals   The federal confidentiality law and regulations set forth some special rules for when a patient's participation in a treatment program is an official condition of probation or parole, sentence, dismissal of charges, release from imprisonment, or other disposition of any criminal proceeding. Although a consent form (or court order) is still required before any disclosure can be made about a criminal justice system referral, the rules concerning duration and revocability of the consent are different (42 C.F.R. 2.22 Title 42 § 2.35). These provisions are designed to streamline as much as possible the ability of the criminal justice system and alcohol and other drug treatment programs to work together, while still ensuring appropriate confidentiality protections.

Specifically, the federal rules state that a consent form that is signed by a client who is mandated into treatment by the criminal justice system can be made irrevocable until a specified date or condition occurs. This is so that an individual who has agreed to enter treatment in lieu of prosecution or punishment cannot then prevent the court or probation, parole, or other agency from monitoring his or her progress.

Furthermore, the rules provide more flexibility in determining the duration of the consent form, stating that duration can be based on a number of factors: the anticipated length of treatment; the type of criminal proceeding; the need for treatment information in disposing of that proceeding; when the final disposition will occur;

and anything else that the patient, program, or criminal justice agency deems pertinent (Id. § 2.35[b]).

Although obtaining a written consent form from the patient is the usual means of authorizing disclosures, the federal confidentiality rules provide a number of other mechanisms for doing so in appropriate circumstances. These are discussed in the following sections.

Court Order

A state or federal court may issue an order that authorizes a program to make a disclosure of patient-identifying information that would otherwise be prohibited. To accomplish their underlying goal of guaranteeing sufficient privacy so that patients will not be afraid to come forward for treatment, however, the federal confidentiality rules permit a court to issue one of these authorizing orders only after following certain procedures and making particular determinations specified by the regulations (42 C.F.R. 2.22 Title 42 §§ 2.63–2.67). In fact—and perhaps most important—a subpoena, search warrant, or arrest warrant, even when it is signed by a judge and says that it is a court order, is not sufficient, when standing alone, to require or even permit a program to make a disclosure (Id. § 2.61). Only a special authorizing order issued pursuant to the federal confidentiality law and regulations enables an alcohol or other drug program to disclose patient information to a court, law enforcement personnel, or anyone else (absent a consent form, of course). This is another major departure from the privacy rules governing other forms of health care records and remains a great source of confusion and consternation for the justice system and alcohol and other drug programs alike. It is also an extremely important protection. Because much alcohol and other drug use is illegal, law enforcement authorities often have much greater interest in records of alcohol and other drug treatment than in any other health care records. The two examples at the beginning of this chapter illuminate that reality. The court order provision in the federal confidentiality rules has served the important function of providing courts the parameters within which they can balance the need for maintaining confidentiality with the need for obtaining information in particular cases and make a reasoned decision that, to the maximum extent possible, satisfies the sometimes competing goals of protecting privacy and seeking justice.

Court-ordered disclosures are sought most often in two types of cases: criminal law and family law (divorces, custody disputes, child neglect, etc.). In criminal cases, an investigative, law enforcement, or prosecutorial agency seeking an order to authorize disclosures for purposes of investigating or prosecuting a patient must meet five stringent criteria:

> 1) The crime involved must be extremely serious, such as an act causing or threatening to cause death or serious injury (but not including possession or sale of illegal drugs); 2) the records sought must be likely to contain information of significance to the investigation or prosecution; 3) there must be no other practical way to obtain the information; 4) the public interest in disclosure must outweigh any actual or potential harm to the patient, the doctor–patient relationship, and the ability of the program to provide services to other patients; and 5) when law enforcement personnel seek the order the program, must have an opportunity to be represented by independent counsel. (Id. § 2.65)

Even if a court decides to issue an order authorizing disclosure for the purpose of investigating or prosecuting patients, the order must limit disclosure and use of the information to those parts of the patient's record that are essential to fulfill the purpose of the order. Under no circumstances may a court authorize a program to turn over the entire patient record to a law enforcement, investigative, or prosecutorial agency. Disclosure must be restricted to those law enforcement and prosecutorial officials responsible for conducting the investigation or prosecution. Use must be limited to investigation of "extremely serious crime or suspected crime specified in the application."

These rules have been very successful in accomplishing their dual goals of protecting both privacy and the pursuit of justice. Courts have issued orders when necessary and denied them when not. As a result, except in a few egregious violations of the law, such as the Fairfax County case, patients have not been scared away from obtaining the life-saving services that benefit them and all of society.

Courts have ordered records disclosed when they constituted important evidence and the other regulatory requirements were satisfied. In *State v. Rollinson* (1987), for example, the court ordered a treatment program to disclose a patient's admissions to several program staff that he had committed a homicide. The court, noting that the information contained in the records was not available elsewhere, ruled that the public interest in disclosure outweighed any possible damage to the treatment relationship.

When the criteria have not been met, however, courts have not hesitated to deny requests for orders authoring disclosures. This especially has been the case when the patient was the victim or another witness to a crime and defendants were seeking access to their treatment records to impeach their credibility. In *United States v. Graham* (1977) and *United States v. Smith* (1986), the U.S. Circuit Courts of Appeals refused to issue orders authorizing disclosure of witnesses' alcoholism and heroin addiction treatment records. Both courts found that, because the witnesses had disclosed their histories of addiction and treatment and could be cross-examined about it, the public interest in maintaining the confidentiality of the records outweighed the defendants' need for the information.

The courts conduct a similar balancing test in family law cases. Thus, in cases such as *In re Romance M* (1993), a custody proceeding in which the court found that treatment records were relevant to the critical question of whether a mother's alcoholism prevented her from properly caring for her children, the courts ordinarily order records disclosed. In cases such as *In re Stephen F.* (1982), however, in which there was no allegation that a father's drug use was the cause of child neglect, the courts often find that any potential value of the records in the proceeding is outweighed by the need to maintain confidentiality.

Child Abuse and Neglect Reporting

As a result of clarifying amendments to the federal confidentiality rules in 1986 and 1987, respectively, the federal confidentiality rules "do not apply to the reporting under state law of incidents of suspected child abuse and neglect to the appropriate state or local authorities" (42 C.F.R. 2.22 Title 42 § 2.12[c][6]). Thus, all alcohol and other drug programs must comply strictly with the provisions of the mandatory child abuse and neglect reporting laws in their states.

However, the exemption for child abuse and neglect reporting applies only to initial reports of child abuse or neglect, not to requests or even subpoenas for additional information or records, even if the records are sought for use in civil or criminal investigations or in proceedings resulting from the program's initial report. In this respect, the federal confidentiality rules treat requests for information related to abuse or neglect that is to be used in court proceedings the same way that they treat other such requests: A court first must issue an appropriate order.

Thus, patient files must still be withheld from child protection agencies absent an appropriate court order or patient consent. Clients are often willing to consent to disclosures to aid investigations of suspected child abuse or neglect, as their refusal to cooperate fully with an investigation may result in loss of custody of their children.

This sensible approach has worked well. Staff of alcohol and other drug programs are able to bring suspected child abuse or neglect to the attention of the appropriate authorities immediately and must do so if they are mandated reporters under state reporting laws. Once those authorities are aware of the situation and begin an investigation, they follow the same rules for obtaining patient records as authorities pursuing any other criminal or civil action.

The legislative history of the 1986 amendment also makes clear that reporting is permitted only when there is a danger of harm to the child, not merely because a parent has abused alcohol or other drugs. This is fortunate because a requirement that all parents who abuse substances be reported could have closed down many treatment programs as word spread that entering treatment would lead directly to a child abuse investigation. Moreover, flooding the child protective system with a multitude of reports that contained no threat or injury to children would retard, not enhance, efforts to combat child abuse.

As Representative Don Edwards (D-CA), Chair of the Judiciary Subcommittee on Civil and Constitutional Rights and one of the authors of the amendment, stated in his speech to the House of Representatives on the legislation,

> The amendment should be applied so it does not dissuade persons from coming forward for drug or alcohol abuse treatment, especially since the children of untreated substance abusers are among the most common victims of child abuse. The amendment is not intended to suggest that substance abuse by itself is a condition that must be reported as child abuse or neglect. As under current practice, there must be some reason to suspect actual or imminent harm to the child. (132 Cong. Rec. H5356, 1986)

Internal Communication

Program staff may disclose information to other staff within the program or to "an entity having direct administrative control over that program" if the recipient needs the information in connection with duties that arise out of the provision of alcohol or other drug abuse diagnosis, treatment, or referral (42 C.F.R. 2.22 Title 42 § 2.12[c][3]). Conversely, staff members who do not need information about particular patients should not have access to it. It is striking—and an illustration of how strenuously the Confidentiality of Records' regulations protect confidentiality—that the drafters saw the need to include this provision. State privilege laws rarely, if ever, limit what information can be disclosed about a patient within a health care facility and instead focus exclusively on disclosures made to outsiders. But when it comes to alcohol and other drug abuse patient records, program staff run afoul of the law if they disclose patient information needlessly to other program staff.

No Patient-Identifying Information

Communications that neither identify an individual as an alcohol or other drug abuser or patient nor verify someone else's identification of the patient are permitted (42 C.F.R. 2.22 Title 42 § 2.12[a][1][i], [e][3]). This is because disclosures that do not identify a patient as having an alcohol or other drug problem do not frustrate the statute's goal of protecting patients from the stigma attached to alcohol and other drug abuse and dependence. The principal ways in which a program may make a "non–patient-identifying disclosure" are by 1) reporting aggregate data about a program's population or some portion of it or 2) communicating information about an individual in a manner that does not disclose that the individual is someone with an alcohol or other drug abuse problem or receiving services from an alcohol or other drug program. Thus, for example, an alcohol or other drug program can reveal how many of its patients have a cocaine problem or are infected with HIV as long as no individual patients are identified directly or indirectly. A hospital or other general health care facility can acknowledge to a patient's family member or friend that she or he has been admitted there as long as it does not reveal the alcohol or other drug problem or diagnosis.

Medical Emergency

Alcohol and other drug programs may make disclosures to medical personnel to the extent necessary to meet a bona fide medical emergency of the patient or any other individual. The regulations define *medical emergency* as a situation that poses an immediate threat to health and requires immediate medical intervention (42 C.F.R. 2.22 Title 42 § 2.51). Both a dangerous drug overdose and attempted suicide would be medical emergencies. Whenever a disclosure is made to cope with a medical emergency, the program must document in the patient's records, the name and affiliation of the recipient of the information, the name of the individual making the disclosure, the date and time of the disclosure, and the nature of the emergency (Id. § 2.51[c]).

Crime at a Program or Against Program Personnel

When a patient has committed or threatened to commit a crime on program premises or against program personnel, the regulations permit the program to report the crime to a law enforcement agency or to seek its assistance. In such a situation, the program can disclose the circumstances of the incident, including the suspect's name, address, last known whereabouts, and status as a patient at the program (42 C.F.R. 2.22 Title 42 § 2.12[c][5]). This provision enables an alcohol or other drug program to take whatever action is necessary—up to and including revealing a patient's identity—to protect its staff, patients, visitors, and property from a patient's illegal activity. While certain provisions must be followed before a program can make disclosures in most other criminal justice contexts, there are no such requirements if a patient commits or threatens a crime against the program or its personnel.

Research or Audits and Evaluations

Scientific Research   The confidentiality regulations permit but do not require a program to disclose patient-identifying information to qualified researchers without patient consent, provided that certain safeguards are met (42 C.F.R. 2.22 Title 42 § 2.52). Researchers must have a protocol that ensures that information will be securely stored and not redisclosed except as allowed by the regulations, and the protocol's confidentiality safeguards must be approved by an independent group of three or more individuals (Id. § 2.52[a]).

Researchers who do receive patient-identifying information are strictly prohibited from redisclosing any patient information to anyone except back to the program. Research reports may not identify a patient, directly or indirectly (Id. § 2.52[b]). Finally, no patient-identifying information may be used to conduct any criminal investigation or prosecution of a patient, even in response to a federal or state court order (Id. § 2.62).

Audits and Evaluations   Government agencies that fund or regulate a program, private agencies that provide financial assistance or third-party payments to a program, and peer-review organizations that review utilization or quality control may have access to program records without patient consent to conduct an audit or evaluation. Any person or organization that conducts an audit or evaluation must agree in writing that it will redisclose patient-identifying information only 1) back to the program, 2) pursuant to a court order to investigate or prosecute the program (not a patient), or 3) to a government agency that is overseeing a Medicare or Medicaid audit or evaluation (42 C.F.R. 2.22 Title 42 § 2.53[c][d]).

The agencies listed in the preceding paragraph may also copy or remove records, but only if they promise in writing to safeguard the confidentiality of patient-identifying information in accordance with the regulations, to redisclose patients' identities only as permitted by the regulations, and to destroy all patient-identifying information when the audit or evaluation is completed (Id. § 2.53[b]). Any other person or organization determined by the program director to be qualified and that pledges in writing to observe the restrictions on redisclosure may also inspect patient records for audit or evaluation purposes without consent, but only the agencies listed in the previous paragraph can be permitted to copy or remove records.

Qualified Service Organization Agreement

Programs may disclose information to a "qualified service organization" without the patient's consent if there is a written agreement between the two in which the service organization

> 1) Acknowledges that in receiving, storing, processing, or otherwise dealing with any information from the program about patients, it is fully bound by the confidentiality regulations; and 2) promises that it will resist, in judicial proceedings if necessary, any efforts to obtain access to information pertaining to patients except as permitted by the regulations. (42 C.F.R. 2.22 Title 42 § 2.12[c][4])

A *service organization* is a person or an agency that provides services to the program, such as data processing; dosage preparation; laboratory analyses; vocational counseling; or legal, medical, accounting, or other professional services (Id. § 2.11). Once the program and the outside agency have entered an agreement of this kind, the program may freely communicate information from patient records to the qualified service organization, but only information that is needed by the organization to provide services to the program.

CONCLUSION

The drafters of the federal law and regulations governing confidentiality of alcohol and other drug patient records took on an enormous challenge: to ensure a sufficient amount of confidentiality so that people who are experiencing what is still one of the most highly stigmatizing illnesses—addiction—will not be afraid to come forward for care, while still enabling the disclosures that are necessary in the modern world. The dramatic achievements of alcohol and other drug treatment and prevention programs are due in no small part to the successful balancing of these important interests embodied in the federal confidentiality rules.

REFERENCES

99th Congress, 2d Sess. (August 4, 1986). Vol. 132 No. 104.
Confidentiality of Records. H.R. Rep. No. 920, 92d Cong., 2d Sess. 33, (1972), *reprinted in* U.S.S.C.A.N. 2072.

In re Commissioner of Social Services v. David R.S., 451 N.Y.S.2d 1 (Ct. App. 1982).
In re Romance M, 622 A.2d 1047 (Conn. Ct. App. 1993).
In re Stephen F., 460 N.Y.S.2d 856 (Fam. Ct. 1982).
Jeanette "A" v. Condon, 728 F. Supp. 204 (S.D.N.Y. 1989).
Masters, B. (1998, August 28). Fairfax police criticized for seizing clinic files. *The Washington Post*, p. C1.
People v. Newman, 32 N.Y.2d 379, 386–387 (1973). New York Court of Appeals.
Legal Action Center. (1996). *Confidentiality: A Guide to the Federal Law and Regulations* (3rd ed.). New York: Author.
State v. Friedman, 1998, Westlaw 170133 (Tenn. Crim. App. April 14, 1998).
State v. Rollinson, 526 A.2d 1283 (Conn. 1987).
United States v. Graham, 548 F.2d 1302 (8th Cir. 1977).
United States v. Smith, 789 F.2d 196 (3d Cir. 1986).
Whyte v. Connecticut Mutual Life Insurance Co., 818 F.2d 1005 (1st Cir. 1987).

10

The Importance of Privacy and Limits to Privacy

John J. Gates and Judy Fitzgerald

As 1999 came to a close, federal law still provided more protection for the privacy of video rental records in the United States than it did for the privacy of medical and mental health records. To many advocates in the health field, this has seemed a perplexing inversion of priorities indicative of a political process in disarray. How else could one explain the swift and relatively unanimous agreement to pass the Video Privacy Protection Act of 1988 (PL 100-618) compared with the protracted debate about a yet-to-be-passed federal law pertaining to some of the most intimate and personal information (i.e., medical and psychiatric records)? What accounts for a Congress that is so ready to agree on the importance of protecting information about video-viewing habits and yet so challenged about a law to protect information about health and illnesses?

The answer may lie in understanding the apparent inversion of priorities as not that at all but rather as the logical result of a political process that is in tune with the time-honored tradition of democratic debate, consumer advocacy, and special-interest lobbying. The Video Privacy Protection Act was passed following the release of the video rental records of Supreme Court nominee Robert Bork. Whether the release of this information had an impact on the eventual rejection of Judge Bork's nomination is not certain. There was, however, strong denunciation by many elected officials and by the press of the use of such "private" information to influence a congressional debate about the suitability of a person to become a member of the highest court in the United States. The release of the information was condemned as an abuse in part because the intent was to harm Bork. Beyond that, there was a collective uneasiness, a group squeamishness resulting from a sense that what had happened to Bork could happen to anyone and that what happened somehow violated the accepted concept of privacy and the feelings of safety and security that are correlated with it. This collective revulsion undoubtedly helped to galvanize the Congress to protect this information for the sake of each citizen as a consumer. What added immeasurably to the success of this consumer protection effort was the support of the video industry. Not only did the owners of video stores ("mom and pop" stores as well as the big chains) support the Video Privacy Protection Act, but so did all others whose business profits related to the rental or sale of videos (producers, distributors, etc.). In the case of video rentals, the privacy interests of the individual consumer and the financial interests of the video industry coincided. It was this convergence of the interests of consumer advocacy and special-interest lobbying that resulted in a political process that was responsive to a united constituency of consumer advocates and special-interest lobbyists rather than a political process in disarray.

The video industry understood that consumers' fears that their private viewing habits becoming public knowledge could result in decreased rentals or sales and hence decreased profits. The same political process was at work when the Congress passed the Electronic Communications Privacy Act of 1986 (PL 99-508) to protect the privacy of consumers' cable television viewing habits. Clearly, there has not been such a convergence of interests in the case of personal health information or of personal financial information.

The history of attempts to safeguard other personally identifying information, including financial information and health information, has been summarized in a report by The Center for Public Integrity (1998) entitled *Nothing Sacred: The Politics of Privacy*. The report makes clear that repeated efforts in the Congress to pass stronger privacy legislation have failed because bills either never made it out of committee or were passed with loopholes. This has been due to opposition to strong legislation by corporate interests. For example, during a 6-year period beginning in 1990, efforts were repeatedly made to update the Fair Credit Reporting Act (PL 104-208). As a result of the easy access to social security numbers (SSNs), thieves were stealing consumer identities, obtaining credit, and leaving victims with a history of bad debt. Consumers were then required to spend, sometimes, years attempting to clear their credit history. Bills were introduced to toughen the law: to require credit bureaus to respond to complaints promptly, to correct errors, and to notify consumers and give them a choice not to have their credit files sold to marketers. The financial services industry (the American Financial Services Association, the Consumer Bankers Association, the American Bankers Association, the National Retail Federation, Visa, and MasterCard) repeatedly lobbied for a weaker bill. As the *Nothing Sacred* report noted, "Not surprisingly, the compromise bill that made its way through Congress in late 1996 contained the 8-year pre-exemption of tougher state laws sought by the industry, and it limited the liability of banks and other creditors that provided incorrect information" (p. 23). The bill also allowed credit bureaus to continue to put together key identifying information about consumers (e.g., name, SSN, mother's maiden name, telephone number, recent addresses) and sell the information to anyone without the permission of the consumer. In effect, the information-sharing practices that had enabled the identity thefts that prompted the reform effort 6 years earlier were allowed to continue, *and* states were preempted to pass any stronger law for 8 years from the passage of the federal law. The question of whether there should be a federal law to protect the privacy of health records that preempts state law, versus the idea that states could pass stronger laws than the federal one, has been a matter of much debate.

An example of industry influence in the health information arena is the proposal to develop a unique personal health identifier to be assigned to each person from birth to death and to be used by all health care providers, insurance companies, payers, and others involved in the delivery and financing of health care. The idea was part of the privacy regulations proposed by the Secretary of the Department of Health and Human Services in 1997, but it had its origin in 1993 as part of Ohio Representative David Hobson's Health Information Modernization and Security Act, essentially designed to simplify health care billing procedures. The Center for Public Integrity stated that "Hobson's idea wasn't really Hobson's idea" (1998, p. 34). The idea was developed and written by a coalition that included the American Health Information Management Association, the American Hospital Association, the American Medical Association, the Association for Electronic Health Care Transactions, Blue Cross and Blue Shield Association, Electronic Data Systems, International Business Machines Corporation, and the Working Group for Electronic Data Exchange. Following its proposal in 1997 and throughout 1998, privacy advocates mounted vigorous opposition to the idea, fearing that the existence of such an identifier posed a great threat to privacy should the number ever get into the wrong hands.

A curious aspect of this debate was that many of the men and women whose organizations favored the unique identifier opposed by the consumer advocates were the same men and women who, as individual providers, have dedicated their lives to caring for those consumers as their patients. What are the issues that prevent a convergence of interests between people whose relationship would ordinarily be based on mutual trust and a common interest in achieving health and overcoming illness? Unlike the protection of video rental records, whereby consumers' wish for privacy was supported by the video industry and no one advocated for access to those records, in the case of health information, significant sectors of the health industry, as well as other sectors of society, have argued for access in opposition to consumers' wish to protect their privacy. It has been this divergence between consumers' interest in keeping their personal health information private and certain societal interests in having access to that health information that has directed debate toward seeking a balance between the privacy of the individual and the legitimate needs of society for access to information. Achieving this balance between competing interests in the health field has been a far more complicated and protracted process for the Congress than was the process of passing the Video Privacy Protection Act. In fact, the Congress has been struggling with this issue off and on for the last quarter of the 20th century. The passage of the Health Insurance Portability and Accountability Act (HIPAA) of 1996 (PL 104-191) has challenged the Congress to resolve some of these privacy issues. It is hoped that this challenge will bring some closure to the effort. The remainder of this chapter comments further on the concept of privacy, explores the various competing interests, and offers recommendations that may help to improve the situation.

IMPORTANCE OF PRIVACY

The idea of personal privacy has a long history and has been considered a right of American citizens but is, as Melton notes in Chapter 4, "notoriously obtuse." Gellman observes in Chapter 7 that "scholarly journals are filled with conflicting theories about the philosophy and purpose of privacy" and suggests that we need not get caught up in those debates. Rather, for practical purposes, he urges focus on the term *data protection* as referring to the collection, maintenance, use, and disclosure of personal information. There is merit to that view, but there is also merit in attempting to understand the following questions: Why do individuals so value their personal privacy? Why do individuals wish to control information about themselves? Why do individuals resist invasions of their privacy?

Hofstadter and Horowitz (1964) reviewed the development of the idea of a right to privacy. An intimation of the idea appeared in approximately A.D. 200 when the portion of the Talmud that summarized the Oral Law of ancient Israel prescribed the minimum distance that a wall opposite a neighbor's windows should be to prevent a man from looking into his neighbor's house. They noted that in Roman law *injuria* meant a willful disregard of another's personality (personhood, personal boundaries, autonomy) and that in Greek law *contumelia* was an infringement on the personality of another. A full exposition of the principle of a right to privacy appeared in the December 15, 1890, issue of the *Harvard Law Review* in an article by Warren and Brandeis (1890, as cited in Hofstadter & Horowitz, 1964). They argued that the right to privacy developed out of the common law principle that individuals should have full protection of their life and property. The right, they argued, had been unrecognized because litigation involving efforts to prevent private letters from being published or personal etchings from being distributed had been characterized as issues of property or contract rights. Warren and Brandeis put forward the idea that more was involved, specifically that common law had secured "to each individual the right of determining, ordinarily, to what extent his thoughts, sentiments, and emotions shall be communicated to others" (Hofstadter & Horowitz, 1964, p. 295). From the legal protection of life and property evolved the recognition of a person's spiritual nature, feelings, and thoughts and the need to protect them.

> The intensity and complexity of life, attendant upon advancing civilization, have rendered necessary some retreat from the world, and man, under the refining influence of culture, has become more sensitive to publicity, so that solitude and privacy have become more essential to the individual; but modern enterprise and invention have, through invasions upon his privacy, subjected him to mental pain and distress, far greater than could be inflicted by mere bodily injury. Nor is the harm wrought by such invasions confined to the suffering of those who may be made the subjects of journalistic or other enterprise. In this, as in other branches of commerce, the supply creates the demand. Each crop of unseemly gossip, thus harvested, becomes the seed of more, and, in direct proportion to its circulation, results in a lowering of social standards and of morality. (Hofstadter & Horowitz, 1964, p. 293)

Concerned by the growing sensationalism of the press of the day and by the threat to privacy posed by the new technology of the "instantaneous photograph," Warren and Brandeis asserted that the underlying principle that protected personal writings (thoughts) and feelings was not that of private property but that of an *inviolate personality.* The term was not defined but seemed to refer to that combination of thoughts, sentiments, and feelings that define the individuality and identity of each person. As Melton notes in Chapter 4, it is that feeling of having been violated that is the common element in our reactions to the following events: being watched while one is undressing; knowing that one's mail has been read; being asked one's income; having one's house entered without permission; having one's purchasing records sold by one company to another; and being required by an employer or a school official to be fingerprinted, provide a urine sample, or take a personality test. The sense of violation derives not from a tangible loss or theft of property or from the humiliation or loss of esteem that may occur in the eyes of others; rather, it is a violation of privacy because these events disturb our own feelings and our *self*-esteem. In this sense, privacy relates to personal dignity, autonomy, personal boundaries, and the development and stability of one's sense of identity. These, in turn, bear on one's relationships with others and the degree to which closeness, trust, social competence, and understanding of social norms develop. Thus, it is not just the individual who is affected by intrusions into privacy but also the social compact on which we must depend to live in civil society.

Warren and Brandeis (1890) recognized that the protection of privacy was needed not only to prevent mental pain and distress to the individual but also to prevent a lowering of social standards and morality. In effect, they argued a public interest in the protection of personal privacy. More than a century later, the Supreme Court supported a psychotherapist privilege for the federal courts in the case of *Jaffee v. Redmond* (1996), thus endorsing the private interest of clients and also affirming that *the mental health of citizens is a public good* of transcendent importance and that the therapist–client privilege facilitates that good by enabling adequate treatment to occur.

Although there still exists no official legal or scientific consensus on why privacy is so valued and why individuals wish to control information about themselves, it is possible to discern some commonly agreed-on ideas. The sense of privacy seems clearly related to one's personal identity, to that continuity of self in a constantly changing world filled with uncertainties and the challenges of change and the comings and goings of loved ones and colleagues and of schools and jobs, and to physical and mental accomplishments and disappointments. The significance of privacy can be identified at an early age. Chapter 4 cites the work of Wolfe (1978) and colleagues, who documented the importance of privacy for children and adolescents in terms of self-esteem, autonomy, and identity formation. It is that sense of self that the child develops, the "me" in the midst of internal and external change, that becomes the foundation of thoughts and feelings and the minor and major choices that individuals make in coping with the inevitable stresses of life. The value of personal privacy thus seems to derive from the need to maintain the integrity of one's sense of self or identity in the interest of effective functioning throughout life. Invasions of privacy are sensed as threats to that sense of self, disruptions to thoughts and feelings and thus to the ability to cope effectively. The protection of privacy is important to prevent harm to such intangibles as "inviolate personality," as Warren and Brandeis put it, or to the maintenance of self-esteem and the development of personal identity as Melton describes in Chapter 4, or the harm from unreasonable searches and seizures of "persons, places, papers, and effects" as covered by the Fourth Amendment to the U.S. Constitution (see Goldman, 1998, for a brief discussion of other relevant amendments). In addition, there are tangible harms that may result if privacy is violated and personal information gets into the wrong hands or is misused. A brief review of some of the tangible harms that might result from the release or misuse of health information follows.

One such potential harm is to an individual's health. With particular reference to therapist–client relationships, privacy is crucial for the development of trust, which in turn fosters honest and candid communications that are so important to successful treatment and, hence, better health and functioning. The patient who believes that his or her privacy will not be protected and whose most intimate and troubling thoughts and feelings will not be kept in confidence by the therapist may not reveal all of the information that ought to be revealed. In some cases, an individual may distort the information out of fear that a third party may obtain access to it, thus providing misleading information to the therapist. In some cases, individuals do not seek the care or help that they need at all. The apparent suicide in 1993 of White House Deputy Counsel Vincent Foster raises the question of whether his not obtaining timely and adequate care was related to his concerns about invasions of privacy and what that might mean to his career. In a speech at The Carter Center in Atlanta, Georgia, in 1996, Pulitzer

Prize–winning author William Styron, who has struggled with depression, reminded his audience that close colleagues of Foster had been aware for months leading up to his suicide that he had lost his appetite (his weight went down 15 pounds), was not sleeping, complained of feeling worthless, and was having difficulty concentrating—all signs of a depressive illness. In trying to understand Foster's fate, Styron said,

> One of the hallmarks of depression is the way it causes victims to magnify troubles out of all proportion to their true measure. Paranoia reigns, harmless murmurs are freighted with menace. Shadows become monsters. Such harassments as Foster endured in Washington could not have been entirely negligible, and they plainly triggered his collapse.
>
> One can understand why he felt betrayed and maligned, why his sense of self-worth may have been compromised. Countless stories have been written since the insinuating *Wall Street Journal* editorials about Foster. The articles claim that he must have feared exposure for some misconduct, probably connected to the Whitewater affair.
>
> Even an anxiety like this rarely leads to thoughts of drastic solutions in the normal mind. Only in someone vulnerable to depression would such worries give rise to the dementia that leads to self-murder. (1996, p. 9)

In Chapter 5 Goin describes the case of "Todd," who refused to give his psychiatrist permission to obtain approval from a managed care company to hospitalize Todd to treat his depression. Todd was afraid that his wife or employer might discover that he had engaged in a homosexual affair. Like Foster, Todd committed suicide. Other patients have simply dropped out of treatment when their therapist has informed them of the need to provide sensitive information to managed care companies, preferring to suffer with their illness than to risk the loss of their privacy. Other surveys have documented public concern about confidentiality in general (Peck, 1994) and the reluctance to talk to one's regular physician about sensitive matters such as HIV/AIDS or substance abuse (Ginsberg et al., 1995).

We must also consider that medical advances contribute to the complexity of privacy concerns, especially in the case of genetic testing. Fear that the results of genetic tests might eventually be used in ways that are adverse to an individual can sometimes dissuade someone from seeking genetic information that may have significant health implications. Sherry, a 38-year-old Navy employee with a young daughter and son, refused to be tested for the genetic mutations that are correlated with many breast and ovarian cancers (Allen, 1998). Despite knowing that her mother and three aunts had experienced breast cancer and that her mother had undergone a prophylactic mastectomy, Sherry refused to obtain the knowledge of her personal situation for fear that once the information was in her medical record (and assuming that the test revealed the presence of the suspect mutations) it might later affect her insurability and employment potential. Sherry's concern about the possible consequences of her personal genetic history not remaining in confidence between her and her physician thus jeopardized her ability to make decisions that would protect her health. These examples make it clear that concerns about privacy not only threaten health but can also threaten life.

Another area of potential tangible harm to individuals is employment. Although the Americans with Disabilities Act (ADA) of 1990 (PL 101-336) prohibits employers from using health care information in making employment decisions, individuals continue to be concerned that they may not be offered a job or be given a promotion or may even be fired because of health information that an employer views negatively. There are good reasons for these continuing concerns. Linowes (1989) found that 35% of the Fortune 500 companies that he surveyed used employees' medical records in making employment-related decisions. Delta Airlines hired Equifax to conduct background checks on thousands of former Pan American Airways employees who were seeking jobs with Delta following the merger of the two companies. It was reported that interviewers asked about drug, alcohol, and financial problems and also about sexual orientation (Anderson, 1991). Patricia Scott charged in her lawsuit that her former employer, Service Employees International Union, fired her when it learned that she had cancer. The Union claimed that they fired her because of poor job performance (Allen, 1998). For most people, the ability to maintain employment or pursue career goals is both the way to make a living and a vital part of their sense of identity and their self-esteem. For people whose identity and self-esteem may have already been battered by their cognitive or affective illness, the fear of not getting a job or losing one looms large.

The inability to obtain health insurance or to afford especially high insurance premiums is another potential tangible harm. Blue Cross of California initially refused to issue a standard health insurance policy for Jacob Turner, a youth whose family had a history of a rare genetic heart disorder (Allen, 1998). Blue Cross relented following the passage of California's genetic antidiscrimination bill, 2 years after Jacob's father applied for the insurance. Concern about the potential misuse of genetic information is also reflected in the fact that 24 states have enacted laws prohibiting health insurers from using genetic information to refuse or limit coverage. In addition, the Human Genome Project has established an Ethical and Legal and Social Implications Program to address the privacy and fair use of genetic information. The relatively rapid legislative responses to the potential harms that may result from the misuse of genetic information indicate the extremely sensitive nature of this issue and the importance that public officials have attached to the protection of genetic information. Our genetic composition represents most closely what is perhaps our "core"—an immutable map of who we are and where we may be going. The fact that it is the most personal and intimate information about us and that the implications of that information apply to each and every human contributed to the speedy consensus toward protection. Despite scientific evidence to the contrary, the prevailing attitude is that the presence of mental illness or substance abuse in the medical record indicates some level of personal weakness—something that happens to "others" (once also the attitude with regard to tuberculosis and cancer, which today seems absurd). Thus, consensus on the nature and degree of privacy protections has been far more elusive.

There is in American society a long tradition that places great importance on the protection of privacy, the safeguarding of personal information (including thoughts and feelings), and the idea that individuals have the right to exercise some degree of choice or control about how and to what degree that information is shared. The tradition is clear that the protection of personal information is important to individual development and identity and that it is also important to society as a whole, significantly linked to our autonomy and liberty as citizens. The tradition is equally clear that there are limits to the protection of privacy in the interest of the public good. The next section summarizes the importance of maintaining societal access to personal information.

IMPORTANCE OF LIMITS TO PRIVACY

Society may enjoy significant benefits from the careful and regulated access to health care information by various sectors of society. Such access is, at times, at odds with society's commitment to the protection of privacy, resulting in the need to balance the protection of personal privacy and the interests of society. As Department of Health and Human Services Secretary Donna E. Shalala stated in her testimony to the Senate Committee on Labor and Human Resources on September 11, 1997, "We must balance our protections of privacy with our public responsibility to support national priorities—public health, research, quality care, and our fight against health care fraud and abuse." The following briefly summarizes these benefits to society.

Quality of Care

Access to both non–personally identifiable and personally identifiable information is critical to society's ability to improve the quality and effectiveness of care now and in the future. Specialists in utilization review, disease management, performance measurement, and research need access to individual cases and to aggregate information to conduct studies that eventually improve the reliability of diagnoses, the effectiveness of treatments, and the education of current and future health care providers. Some privacy advocates have argued that patients should have the opportunity to give their informed consent or refuse to give their consent to the release of personally identifiable information to these various specialists. The alternative point of view is that relatively unrestricted access to non–personally identifiable information is necessary in the interest of efficiency of procedures and to ensure that reviews and studies are based on data that are representative of the entire population being served. In effect, there is concern that, if consumers have the opportunity to refuse to allow their information to be utilized for review or research purposes, the data on which studies are conducted will be biased, thus adversely affecting the validity of findings.

Further supporting the idea that personally identifiable information might be made available to researchers without patient consent is a proposal that such release occur only when there has been a determination by an Institutional Review Board (IRB) that the research would involve minimal risk to participants, and that the absence of consent would not adversely affect the rights or welfare of participants, and that it would not be practical to conduct the research if consent were required. The researcher would also be required to ensure that personally identifiable information would be eliminated as soon as possible and that safeguards would be put in place to protect the unauthorized disclosure of such information. It should be noted that researchers have indeed had this sort of access to information for many years and that most have responsibly protected personal information. Improvements in medical care over the last several decades speak to the value of maintaining access to health information for review, evaluation, and research purposes. Occasionally, however, violations of privacy have occurred in the past and likely will occur in the future, reinforcing the need for clear guidelines and vigilant monitoring of compliance.

Public Health

The health of individuals and of the population as a whole can be enhanced if public health officials at local, state, and national levels have access to health care information. The potential to prevent disease and premature death and to promote health can be enhanced when public health authorities undertake surveillance and epidemiological research, collect information, and provide reports on disease patterns and the health status of the population. Actions taken by public health authorities historically have been based on a vast and coordinated data collection, analysis, and reporting system and have resulted in the reduction of many infectious diseases, the containment of periodic outbreaks of disease as a result of microorganism contamination of food or water, and the containment of sexually transmitted diseases. These successes have been possible even though state laws govern public health reporting requirements and even though there are significant differences from state to state. It is also significant to note that although much of the information utilized by public health authorities is not personally identifiable, a considerable amount of information is necessarily personally identifiable (e.g., for the reporting and containment of sexually transmitted diseases including HIV/AIDS). This is information of the most intimate kind with great potential for embarrassment and discrimination to the subject of the information if improperly used or disclosed. It is fair to say that public health authorities have an outstanding track record of having secured the confidentiality of this information. Even with such a record, larger electronic databases and the wide variability among the states in terms of regulations regarding the storage of, access to, and use of information necessitated the creation of the Model State Public Health Privacy Project. The aim of this project is to put forward a model *state* law that would, if adopted, improve the protection of confidential, personally identifiable information held by public health departments while at the same time facilitating a national reporting system, especially regarding HIV/AIDS information (Gostin & Hodge, 1998). Historically, informed consent by consumers has not been necessary for information to be made available to public health authorities, and there has not been any serious proposal put forward during recent discussions regarding privacy and confidentiality legislation to do so.

Protecting Others from Harm

There are certain circumstances in which legislative and judicial bodies have required that information be made available to individuals or agencies to protect individuals from harm. Health care providers are obligated to inform public health officials of individuals who have a sexually transmitted disease so that public health officials can work with the infected individuals to identify sexual partners to reduce the spread of the disease. Health care providers are also required to report suspected cases of child abuse or neglect to appropriate state child protection or welfare agencies so that they in turn can investigate the suspicions to determine whether abuse or neglect is occurring and take appropriate actions to protect the interests of the child. Courts may also order the release of certain information when it is pertinent to certain civil proceedings (e.g., divorce, child custody) or to criminal prosecutions. For obvious reasons, in none of the previous instances is the consent of the consumer required. In the case of a person who is experiencing a mental illness who may, in the course of therapy, reveal to his or her counselor a serious intent to harm another individual and the counselor judges that there is a likelihood that the patient may actually follow up on the intent, the courts have ruled that the therapist has a duty to warn the individual threatened or to alert appropriate law enforcement officials of the possibility of harm (*Tarasoff v. Regents of University of California,* 1976).

The previous examples illustrate limitations on the right to privacy that have been broadly accepted in society. The various court decisions and laws that have been passed to ensure access to these kinds of health care information reflect a pervasive societal view that the protection from harm to others is a legitimate reason for limiting the right to privacy. At the same time, there has been an expectation that those who have access to such information must use that information responsibly and after careful consideration of the accuracy of the information and with due regard to limiting its disclosure only to those who need to know. The investigation of suspicions of child abuse or neglect, for example, must be pursued with the primary goal of safeguarding the child but also with an awareness of potential adverse impact on parents, caregivers, and the family unit. Patients who reveal thoughts or fantasies involving harm to other individuals may or may not act on them. The therapist's duty to warn these other individuals requires the therapist to make a difficult judgment of whether to share that information outside the therapeutic relationship, knowing that to do so may have severe consequences on the trust involved in the therapist–client relationship.

Containing Costs and Preventing Fraud

Access to certain health care information by payers (private and public), claims processors, and insurance and managed care companies can result in containment of health care costs, a potential benefit to consumers who pay for care either through insurance premiums or out of their own pocket, to employers who pay for a significant portion of health care benefits, and to taxpayers whose taxes support government-subsidized health care such as provided through the Medicaid and Medicare programs. When provided with the necessary information, electronic billing and payment mechanisms have the potential to achieve great efficiencies to the administrative overhead associated with health care provision. The increasing automation of such information also has the potential to enable officials to prevent and detect fraud. It has been estimated that 10% of all health care expenditures are the result of inefficiency and waste or outright fraud. The containment of unnecessary costs thus can make health care more affordable and result in more accessible care for more people.

Concerns have been expressed both about the numbers of administrative and fiscal personnel with access to health care information and about exactly how much and what kind of information such individuals need to have. Consequently, there has been discussion of the need for guidelines to reduce the number of individuals who have access and to specify a minimal data set necessary for financial and administrative transactions. This is clearly a desirable goal. However, the subtle nuances of the privacy debate are most visible in the attempt to define the gray areas of a "legitimate need for access" to an individual's health information.

Access by Family Members and Law Enforcement Officials

There appears to be some level of public consensus on the value of the societal benefits derived from improving the quality of care, safeguarding public health, protecting individuals from harm, containing costs, and preventing fraud. Certain other requests for access do not have the same degree of public consensus and require a careful weighing of pros and cons to determine the optimal balance of individual protection and the public good. Two such areas that have generated significant controversy are the needs for access to information by family members and by law enforcement officials.

In Chapter 3, Lefley argues that family education in the medical sector is standard practice; however, "in the psychiatric sector, despite a dozen rigorous studies showing the benefits to the patient of family education, families continue to receive little information and almost no formal training in illness management." This is especially challenging because, as Lefley reports, "it is estimated that, on average, 50% of people with severe mental illness live at home with family caregivers." Family members' desire to fulfill their roles as caregivers is, at times, at odds with consumers' wishes to control the release of information. A number of states have attempted to identify a middle ground, specifying types of information that can be released to family members without client consent. However, the diverse range of viewpoints and practices of individual professionals regarding the release of information to family members has led to inconsistent application of rules, often resulting in feelings of frustration and confusion for well-intentioned family members.

Access to health information by law enforcement officials represents one of the most controversial aspects of the privacy debate. In cases in which a clear and direct threat to the well-being of another individual exists, the law is clear in protecting the safety of those involved. A concern exists, however, that law enforcement officials may hide behind the guise of "case investigation" in the pursuit of information that would otherwise not be available to them.

While opposing groups might equally value the public safety protection offered by law enforcement agencies, perceptions vary widely regarding the amount and nature of information that should be made available to law enforcement personnel. Fears about "Big Brother" incite a collective uneasiness about unfettered access. At the same time, fears about guilty criminals walking the streets demand that we think carefully about barriers to criminal investigations.

Access by both family members and law enforcement personnel requires that careful consideration be given to the opposing ends of the opinion spectrum. As in each aspect of the debate, a test of reasonableness must be employed consistently. By focusing on the goal of reasonableness and balance and by enforcing standards that are implemented at every level, a compromise is feasible.

Given the important benefits to the public good and that achieving these benefits must be balanced with the individual and societal benefits that result from the protection of personal privacy, there are a number of complex issues that must be addressed. The last section of this chapter discusses these issues on the premise that we may do the best job possible by keeping in mind that all of society derives benefits from *both* the protection of privacy *and* the reasonable and guided intrusion to some extent into that privacy. Society does not derive benefits from one or the other but from the appropriate balance of both. The occasional argument that emphasizes oppositional interests may not serve society as well in addressing privacy concerns.

OPTIONS AND ISSUES

Basically, three legislative options have been discussed in addressing privacy and confidentiality:

1. Establish a federal law that preempts state laws and sets a high standard of information management practices with which all would have to comply. This federal law would be similar to the federal substance abuse law, in effect creating a "ceiling." (It should be noted that the federal substance abuse law does allow states to establish more stringent requirements for disclosure of information, but almost all states have continued to view the federal law as stringent enough.)
2. Establish a federal law that provides minimum requirements with which all would have to comply but that would not preempt state laws that contained stronger or more stringent information management practices. Most bills introduced in the Congress in 1997 and 1998 were of this type. Such a law, if enacted, would create a "floor."
3. Establish guidelines for a model state law that would not be binding on any jurisdiction but that would enable state legislators to understand better the core issues to consider in drafting a state law. Petrila has outlined such an approach for a model mental health law in Chapter 6.

Details vary, but all three options have included similar elements, such as informed consent, criteria for disclosure and redisclosure, diverse recipients of information, types and amounts of information to disclose, access by consumers to their own records and opportunity to correct errors, and penalties for violations. Given these similarities, is there any advantage of one option compared with the others in terms of reaping the benefits of both the protection of personal privacy and the guided intrusion into that privacy? More specific, which option might better protect privacy and confidentiality, allow reasonable access to certain information that serves the public good, help to contain costs through administrative efficiencies, and protect others from harm? It is suggested here that a federal law that contains strong protections for privacy and that preempts state laws (i.e., a federal law that sets a ceiling, or high standard) might have advantages over the other two options. This suggestion is based on both the success of the federal substance abuse law and the uniformity or standardization made possible by such a law.

The variation in state laws that govern the confidentiality of health information has led scholars such as Gellman and Petrila to conclude that there is very little consistent protection available to consumers. It is instructive to look at the summary of state laws regarding mental health records in the appendix at the end of this book to see the variations in terms of definitions, access to records by consumers and others, ability to correct erroneous information, those covered by the laws, and so forth. Not only do these variations result in inconsistent protection for consumers, but they also present challenges to the efficient transmission of information between states, thus increasing administrative costs among national managed care companies, large networks of health care providers, and national companies involved in the processing of health care claims. A strong federal law, one that sets a ceiling rather than a floor, governing all health care information would have several advantages over the existing patchwork of state laws, a model state law, or a weak federal law that sets a floor. These advantages include the potential to satisfy virtually all consumer protection advocates, to eliminate the inefficiencies and extra costs that result from the necessity to alter business practices to accommodate 50 different jurisdictions, to avoid potentially expensive and lengthy debate and litigation over which laws or portions of laws are stronger or weaker, and to continue to provide appropriate access to information for those sectors of society with legitimate reasons for access.

An additional factor that should be considered is the privacy directive set forth by the European Union. As we acknowledge that health care has become national, so should we recognize the likelihood that it will become more global, with increasing exchanges of clinical, research, administrative, and fiscal databases. The European Union's law sets conditions for the international transfer of personal information from the European Union to nonmember countries. The directive prohibits transfers of information to any country that fails to ensure an adequate level of protection to health information. The lack of a clear, strong standard in the United States could soon become a barrier to the international exchange of health care information.

A good case can be made for the view that the federal substance abuse law has been successful. Samuels concludes Chapter 9 by observing the following:

The drafters of the federal law and regulations governing confidentiality of alcohol and drug patient records took on an enormous challenge: to ensure a sufficient amount of confidentiality so that people experiencing what is still one of the most highly stigmatizing illnesses—addiction—will not be afraid to come forward for care, while still enabling the disclosures that are necessary in the modern world. The dramatic achievements of alcohol and other drug treatment and prevention programs in the past two decades are due in no small part to the successful balancing of these important interests embodied in the federal confidentiality rules.

In effect, people came for treatment, privacy and confidentiality were well protected, providers were paid, fraud was investigated, and law enforcement and the courts got the information they needed. Although the federal substance abuse law applied only to federally assisted programs, its success appears to support further exploration of a federal law similar in design that would apply to all health care information. It may be that, in the details of its design and implementation, we find a closer convergence between the interests of the individual patients/consumers and the interests of others to have access to certain personal information about those patients/consumers.

Chapter 9 contains the elements of the federal substance abuse law that arguably have made it the strongest law in terms of the protection of privacy and confidentiality while still permitting disclosures of information that serve various societal needs. Should there develop interest in a similar law governing *all* health information, many of the same elements would need to be included. Four of the most important of these elements are the special treatment of sensitive information, limiting the amount and type of information disclosed, informed consent, and accountability for all. Each is discussed briefly to address some of the questions that might arise under any legislative option.

Special Treatment of Sensitive Information

Some mental health advocates have urged that mental health information should receive the same kind of sensitive special treatment now afforded to substance abuse information. This proposal raises a double-edged sword. On the one hand, the long history of stigma and discrimination experienced by people with mental illness would seem to argue for special treatment of the information. On the other hand, there is a concern that identifying mental health information as distinct and separate from overall health information merely reinforces the stigma that exists. The same dilemma exists for HIV/AIDS and for genetic information. However, the dilemma would be significantly resolved if the law set a very high standard for information management similar to the federal substance abuse law and if this new law applied to all health information.

As the next section discusses, there may still be good reason to differentiate among types of information in personal records, but its "sensitive nature" need not be one of them if all health information were afforded maximum confidentiality. Treating all information similarly might, over time, help to reduce the stigma now associated with certain disorders, such as mental illness.

Limiting the Amount and Type of Information Disclosed

The increase in the number of third-party reviewers and data management, fiscal, and other administrative personnel has generated increased concerns about the numbers of individuals wanting access to personal health care information and about the types of information to which they want access. In response to these concerns, there has been growing interest in limiting the number of people who have access and in developing guidelines that would make clearer which information should be disclosed to which entities (individuals or organizations) for which purposes and for how long. It has been recommended that guidelines be developed to specify the amount and type of information needed for payment purposes, for research, and for treatment. Guidelines for special populations also could be developed. For example, it has been recommended that special guidelines regarding informed consent be developed for children and adolescents, taking into account their developmental stages and particularly addressing information to be shared with parents. Melton suggests in Chapter 4 that a model interagency agreement be developed in view of the many agencies that are interested in children's services and the difficulties encountered in sharing information because of different rules and regulations.

The development of guidelines regarding which information would be released to which individuals or organizations for which purposes would enable the creation in the health information record of what has been referred to as *zones of privacy* or *tiers of confidentiality*. Such zones or tiers can make relatively clear distinctions among different kinds of information. Intimate, clinical details revealed in psychotherapy sessions, for example, might remain in one zone or tier and be available only to health care providers, whereas diagnostic and basic treatment information might be made available to payers. Modern computer security technology makes this feasible. The more challenging part will be classifying information into categories and resisting the temptation to place too much information in the most confidential tier or, alternatively, not to put enough information there.

In clarifying which information could be disclosed to whom, such guidelines might

1. Reduce the number of recipients of information (there seems an inherent value in limiting the number of people who have access to the minimum possible—authorized users misuse information as much as or more than unauthorized users)
2. Ensure that recipients receive the information necessary for them to perform their functions (e.g., pay bills, review care, conduct research) but no more than what is necessary
3. Specify limitations on redisclosure of information
4. Enable all consumers to understand clearly the intended uses of their personal health information

Consideration might also be given to codifying these guidelines as agency regulations.

Informed Consent

If the violation of privacy is sensed as a threat to the identity and self-esteem of people without cognitive or emotional problems, then such a violation can be even more threatening to people whose cognitive or emotional problems have already compromised their sense of identity and self-esteem. Anxiety, depression, uncertainty, and confusion already complicate the lives of such individuals. The therapist–client relationship has as its goal the amelioration of these difficulties, not the compounding of them; thus, the relationship must develop in a context of caring, mutual respect, and trust that what is shared will be protected in support of the client's well-being. These characteristics of a sound therapeutic relationship do not necessarily require an absolute protection against sharing certain information with certain others for certain purposes, but it does seem important to such a relationship that the client know in advance of providing information to third parties which information is to be given, to whom, and for what purposes and that the client have the opportunity to consent to the release of that information.

It is clear from the previous chapters that there is not agreement on whether the release of any and all information should require client consent. Some have argued that *informed consent* should always be obtained from clients prior to releasing any information, whereas others have argued that that would be inefficient and increase the cost of care. The latter argue that the release of specific information to specific parties should be predicated on the notion of *presumed consent,* indicating a general agreement that all disclosures deemed necessary in the pursuit of payment and treatment can occur without additional approval. There may be public consensus regarding the efficiency impact of presumed consent, and most probably also would acknowledge that most Americans have regularly signed standardized consent forms for years in their doctors' offices and in hospitals and often have done so without reading all of the small print, implying that presumed consent is a de facto element of health care information practices. However, the proponents of informed consent argue that even a perfunctory practice that offers individuals the opportunity to exercise choice about the sharing of personal information is important to the sense of protection of personal identity.

The articulation and enforcement of a few basic principles might go a long way in improving the current approach to informed consent. People have a right to know how their information is being used, a right to a grievance procedure if they wish to challenge the accuracy of the information in the record, and a right to expect that individuals who misuse their information will be held accountable. The elements to be incorporated into privacy guidelines should therefore include the following requirements:

1. A commonsense consent form that can be readily explained and understood, describing which information will be released to whom and for what purpose
2. That the entity disclosing the information will keep an audit trail that indicates where the information has been sent and that this audit trail will be available to a consumer on request
3. A grievance procedure and appeal mechanism to challenge the accuracy of the information contained in the record
4. That the entity disclosing the information will also provide strict guidelines for redisclosure and identify penalties for violations

In Chapter 2, Campbell points out that for people with mental illness, special consideration must be given to the competence of the patient to give consent and to the extent to which subtle or not-so-subtle coercion is used to induce consent. There are also special considerations when a person has been referred involuntarily, pursuant to a civil commitment procedure, for evaluation and treatment.

Accountability for All

Historically, physicians have been bound by both a code of ethics and state laws to protect the privacy of health care information about their patients. Unfortunately, although most states have laws that pertain to physicians, there are fewer that address other health care providers and only a handful of states bind insurers. Now that so many individuals have access to health care information, there has emerged the concept of a "health information trustee" (i.e., the idea that any person who has access to health care information should be held responsible for the proper handling and protection of that health care information). Thus, all types of health care providers, as well as third-party reviewers and claims processing and administrative personnel, would be subject to civil and criminal penalties for violations of laws or regulations. Organizational commitment to policy development, training of all staff, and monitoring of compliance can achieve a high standard of protection of privacy.

If adopted in law and policy, the concept of uniform accountability for violations of privacy regulations would go a long way toward reducing the unauthorized disclosure of information and its misuse. This would also require the development of guidelines regarding redisclosure (or secondary disclosure) of information, which historically has been a major way in which health care information has been inappropriately released or misused. The notion here is that any time individuals or organizations receive health care information, they also would receive redisclosure guidelines, which would make clear the penalties for their violation. The Model State Public Health Privacy Project, for example, has considered a fine of $5,000 and up to 1 year in jail for negligently violating confidentiality and a fine not to exceed $50,000 and up to 5 years in jail for the intentional violation with an intent to profit or cause malicious harm.

CONCLUSION

It is important to acknowledge that despite the apparent advantages that might result from a strong federal law, there has not been widespread support for one for at least two reasons. First, since the beginning of the administration of President Ronald Reagan in 1981, the Congress and state legislators have consistently voted for more state and local control over a broad array of matters and less control by the federal government. The notion of a strong federal law that would preempt state laws would be counter to this longstanding political dynamic. The seeming paradox of a broad coalition in support of a weak federal law is understandable by noting the benefit to commercial interests of the standardization of the storage, transmission, and management of information if the law also allows for the automatic release of certain information, especially to payers. The second reason for the lack of significant support for a strong federal law is the absence of the broad groundswell of fear and concern generated by the violent criminal activity associated with the alcohol and other drug problem. Although there has been public concern about the spread of HIV/AIDS and about the occasional dangerous behavior of some people with mental illness, the fact that the Congress has *not* passed a strong federal law indicates that they have not felt pressure from a broad constituency similar to that associated with addictive disorders.

The development and use of computer technology have increased concerns about protecting personal privacy. The technology will continue to evolve, and it will be used and prompt us, as it already has, to develop technological, legal, and policy safeguards to prevent its misuse. If history is a guide, then it is likely that the technological changes (e.g., faster, bigger, more secure computers and better, more effective ways to breach that security) will occur faster than changes in laws and policies. Society must be motivated to adjust those laws and policies to maintain the balance between personal privacy and society's needs to limit that privacy—and, hence, to derive benefits from both. However, there are powerful, well-organized, and well-funded forces that favor more and more access to personal information, and many would agree that the privacy of Americans has eroded. Some would argue that consumer advocates, who are not as well organized or funded, have been losing ground.

Despite the likelihood of formidable opposition to a strong federal law, HIPAA has provided a window of opportunity for thoughtful, informed decision making on privacy at the federal level. Although a ceiling seems to provide the most significant benefits, there will be costs involved and such costs should be well researched and considered. However, the state-by-state patchwork approach is no longer viable. It does not afford a minimum level of consistent protection that Americans have a right to expect and often mistakenly assume that they already have. Uniform standards should be the minimum requirement, and setting these standards at the highest level is a lofty but achievable goal. Even if movement toward this goal were to occur through a protracted phase-in process, it would represent significant progress for the protection of privacy for all, particularly for some of our most vulnerable citizens. The combination of a high standard of privacy protection and uniformity of health information practices that would be possible with a strong federal law has the potential to overcome the historic divergence of interests between individual consumers and others interested in access to personal information.

Gellman observes in Chapter 7 that the Supreme Court looks to individual and societal expectations about privacy to help interpret the Constitution and its amendments and that familiarity with technology can have an impact on our expectations for privacy. "Once everyone is used to technology, it grows more difficult to argue that the technology violates expectations of privacy." His conclusion is that legislation is needed to protect the erosion of privacy expectations. The challenge is how to level the lobbying playing field between the large, well-organized, and well-funded stakeholders and the less-organized and less-funded consumer protectionists so that the legislation indeed provides the protections to which Gellman refers. Perhaps Campbell's ideas of person-driven, people-first systems of health information management, guided by principles that are based on the value of individual consumers, would be a step toward leveling the lobbying playing field. Legislation that is based on such values might incorporate requirements for the participation of individual consumers in health policy development in both the private and public sectors; the development and tracking of compliance with laws, regulations, and policies; the success of enforcement mechanisms; and the development and dissemination of reports regarding privacy and confidentiality (perhaps as a portion of a "report card" in the section on consumer satisfaction). Above all, legislative and policy efforts must be mindful of the fact that when we consider privacy of the health record, human lives and livelihoods are at stake. The golden rule of treating others the way you wish to be treated may be sage advice to offer those who will shape the privacy decision-making process.

REFERENCES

Allen, A. (1998, February 8). Exposed. *Washington Post Magazine,* p. W10.

Americans with Disabilities Act (ADA) of 1990, PL 101-336, 42 U.S.C. §§ 12101 *et seq.*

Anderson, J.R. (1991, December 9). No one cares if it's true: Background checks have little limit. *Newsday,* p. 6.

The Center for Public Integrity. (1998). *Nothing sacred: The politics of privacy.* Washington, DC: Author.

Electronic Communications Privacy Act of 1986, PL 99-508, 18 U.S.C.S. § 2510.

Fair Credit Reporting Act of 1996, PL 104-208, 15 U.S.C.S. § 1692.

Ginsberg, K.R., Slap, G.B., Cnaan, A., Forke, C.M., Balsley, C.M., & Rouselle, D.M. (1995). Adolescents' perceptions of factors affecting their decision to seek health care. *Journal of the American Medical Association, 273,* 191–198.

Goldman, J. (1998). Privacy in health information: A legal framework. In *Protecting the confidentiality of patient information in a rapidly changing health care system: Summary of a national conference* (Appendix E, pp. 1–10). Washington, DC: Health Systems Research, Inc.

Gostin, L., & Hodge, J., Jr. (1998). *Model State Public Health Privacy Project: Privacy and security of public health information with specific emphasis on HIV/AIDS* [On-line]. Available: http://www.critpath.org/msphpa/privacy.htm

Health Insurance Portability and Accountability Act of 1996, PL 104-191, 42 U.S.C. §§ *Health Insurance Portability and Accountability Act: Hearings Before the Senate Committee on Labor and Human Resources* 105th Cong., 2nd Sess. (1997) (testimony of D.E. Shalala, Secretary, U.S. Department of Health and Human Services).

Hofstadter, S.H., & Horowitz, G. (1964). *The right of privacy.* New York: Central Book Company.

Jaffee v. Redmond, 518 U.S.1 (1996).

Linowes, D. (1989). *Privacy in America; Is your private life in the public eye?* Urbana: University of Illinois Press.

Peck, R. (1994). Results from an Equifax poll; on concerns about medical confidentiality. *Medical and Health News, 14,* 10.

Styron, W. (1996). Once again, behold the stars. In *The Report of the Second Annual Rosalynn Carter Georgia Mental Health Forum* (pp. 6–9). Atlanta: The Carter Center.

Tarasoff v. Regents of University of California, 551 P.2d 334 (1976).

Video Privacy Protection Act of 1988, PL 106-628, 18 U.S.C. § 2710.

Wolfe, M. (1978). Childhood and privacy. In I. Altman & J. Wohlwill (Eds.), *Human behavior and environment: Vol. 3. Advances in theory and research* (pp. 175–222). New York: Plenum.

Appendix

State Mental Health
Confidentiality Law Provisions

John Petrila

This table provides information regarding key provisions of the statutes of the 50 states and the District of Columbia regarding the confidentiality of mental health information. The table provides the following information.

The first column (State) provides the name of the state and the reference to the relevant mental health law provisions. In the case of a few states, particularly those without a discrete mental health confidentiality law, the citation to the statute that governs general health care confidentiality is provided. For a handful of states, both the mental health confidentiality law and the general confidentiality law are provided because both apply to mental health records. In those cases, the mental health reference is designated by (mh), whereas the general provision is marked (general).

The second column (Mental health law?), which is divided into two subcolumns (Yes and No), notes whether a state has a separate statute addressing the confidentiality of mental health records.

The third column (Consent form detailed?) notes whether the state law spells out requirements for a consent form.

The fourth column (Provider access?) notes whether the state law specifically addresses the release of information to other treatment providers. If the column is marked with an X, then the state law permits release to other providers without consent of the patient. If the column is blank, then the statute does not address the issue. If explanatory material is provided, then it means that release is permitted with conditions (e.g., patient consent).

The fifth column (Payer access?) provides information on whether and how the state law addresses the release of information to other payers or providers of other benefits.

The sixth column (Danger to third party or self?) shows how the state *statute* handles the issue of releasing information in situations in which a third party (or the client) might be endangered by the client. Note that this does not provide information about court rulings that might create an obligation in a particular state; the point of this analysis is to show what state statutes cover, because statutory reform is the subject of most of the debates regarding confidentiality. It is therefore possible that a court ruling might address this topic even though the statute does not.

The seventh column (Law enforcement access?) describes what the mental health law permits in terms of release of information to law enforcement officials. As the table suggests, most state laws address situations in which a patient might be missing from a treatment facility. National reform proposals also focus on efforts to address fraud, an issue addressed by only a few states.

The eighth column (Client access?) examines client access to information. The phrase "absent harm" describes statutory provisions that permit access unless a clinician determines that access might present a potential harm to the client.

The ninth column (Family access?) details the access of families to client information. States that provide access typically limit it to families who are acting as caregivers and limit the type of information to prognosis, diagnosis, medications, and a summary of the treatment plan. Whether client consent is required is noted as well.

The table does not provide information on access by researchers, public health officials, and oversight agencies. As Chapter 6 notes, states almost universally provide unconsented access to records in these circumstances if certain conditions are met (e.g., in the case of research, the approval of an Institutional Review Board). As the text also notes, at least some reform proposals would tighten access in some of these circumstances. However, for the purposes of this table, given the virtual unanimity among the states, these issues are not covered.

The information in this table is current through August 1998.

State mental health confidentiality law provisions

State	Mental health law? Yes	Mental health law? No	Consent form detailed?	Provider access?	Payer access?	Danger to third party or self?	Law enforcement access?	Client access?	Family access?
Alabama Ala. Code §22-50-62 (1975)	X								
Alaska Alaska Stat. §47.30.845 (1996)	X			X			if patient absent without consent or imminent danger to community		
Arizona Ariz. Rev. Stat. Ann. §36-509 (1993)	X			X		explicit threat to third party (36-517.02)	if patient absent without consent	provider may limit access (36-507)	family involved in care; limited to prognosis, diagnosis, and medication; no consent
Arkansas Ark. Code Ann. §20-46-103, 20-46-104 (1991)	X								

(continued)

State mental health confidentiality law provisions *(continued)*

State	Mental health law? Yes	Mental health law? No	Consent form detailed?	Provider access?	Payer access?	Danger to third party or self?	Law enforcement access?	Client access?	Family access?
California Cal. [Welfare and Inst.] Code §5328 (West 1998)	X			X	to extent necessary to make a claim	serious danger to reasonably foreseeable victim	protect officials and examiner; third parties; court can order if crime by patient who is a sex offender (5328.01)		with patient consent (5328.1)
Colorado Col. Rev. Stat. Ann. §27-10-120 (West 1990)	X			X	to extent necessary to make claims			yes, unless negative impact on patient (25-1-801)	location and fact of admission; patient consent to prognosis, diagnosis, medications, side effects (27-10-120.5)
Connecticut Conn. Gen. Stat. Ann. §52-146f (privilege statute) (West 1991)		X		X	limited info. to agencies involved in fee collection	risk of imminent physical injury to self or others		yes, unless harm to patient (20-7C)	

State / Citation								
Delaware Del. Code Ann. title 16 §5161 (13) (1995)	X							yes, absent harm to patient
District of Columbia D.C. Code Ann. §6-2004-6-2026 (1995)	X		X (6-2012)	limited info (6-2017)	protect client or another from imminent harm (6-2023)	if third party endangered		in emergency (6-2023)
Florida Fla. Stat. Ann. 14 §394.4615 (West Supp. 1998)	X			X	intent to harm third party (394.4615; 455.2415)		absent harm to patient	patient or next of kin may obtain treatment plan summary; current condition
Georgia Ga. Code Ann. §37-3-166 (1995)	X			X		reveal whether individual is a patient	yes, absent harm (33-3-167)	
Hawaii Haw. Rev. Stat. §334-5 (1996)	X						yes, absent harm (622-57)	
Idaho (hospital record privilege 39-1392b)		X						

(continued)

State mental health confidentiality law provisions *(continued)*

State	Mental health law? Yes	Mental health law? No	Consent form detailed?	Provider access?	Payer access?	Danger to third party or self?	Law enforcement access?	Client access?	Family access?
Illinois Ill. Ann. Stat. Ch. 740 para. 110/2 - 110/17 (Smith-Hurd 1998)	X		X (110/5)	with consent unless patient incompetent or unavailable (110/6)		clear risk to client or others; secret service or state police (110/2)		no limits (110/4)	
Indiana Ind. Code Ann. §16-39-2-1– 16-39-4-6 (West Supp. 1998)	X		X	to obtain payment; managed care providers (16-39-2-6)		harm to self or others (16-39-2-6)	escape; risk to patient or third party; crime on premises; Secret Service (16-39-2-6)	yes, unless harm (16-39-2-4)	
Iowa Iowa Code Ann. §228.1–228.9 (West Supp. 1998)	X		X (228.3)	X	to collect fees (228.5); to payers with consent (228.7)				limited info; notice to client (228.8)
Kansas Kan. Stat. Ann. §65-5601– 65-5605 (1992; 1997 Supp.)	X			treatment facilities (65-5603)	any info relevant to the collection of a bill (65-5603)	protect identified third party (65-5603)		yes, unless harm (65-5603)	

Kentucky	X			identifiable victim (Ky. Rev. Stat. Ann. §202 A.400 [Michie 1998]		yes, on written request (Ky. Rev. Stat. Ann. §422.317 [Michie 1998]	
Louisiana	X						
Maine Me. Rev. Stat. Ann. title 34-B1207 (West 1964; 1997–1998 Supp.)	X		to obtain payment	danger to evaluator or others		yes, absent harm (1711-B)	client consent; some limits
Maryland Md. Code Ann. 4-307 (Michie Supp. 1997)	X	client consent	yes (4-305)	specified victim (5-609)	absent without consent; danger to third party (5-609)		
Massachusetts Mass. Ann. Laws Ch. 123-36 (dept. records); Ch. 112-129A; 135A (privilege) (Lawyers Cooperative Publishing 1998)	X		access under privilege statute (129A[5]; 135A)	identifiable victim (123-36B)			

(continued)

State mental health confidentiality law provisions *(continued)*

State	Mental health law? Yes	Mental health law? No	Consent form detailed?	Provider access?	Payer access?	Danger to third party or self?	Law enforcement access?	Client access?	Family access?
Michigan Mich. Comp. Laws Ann. §330-1748–330. 1750 (West Supp. 1998)	X			with patient consent or to prevent harm	to apply for or receive benefits	prevent harm to client or others		unless legally incompetent	
Minnesota Minn. Stat. Ann. §144.335 (West 1998)		X		other providers in the health care entity or with patient consent	patient consent			yes, absent harm	patient consent
Mississippi Miss. Code Ann. §41-21-97 (1972)	X			yes	eligibility for benefits	identifiable victim	identifiable victim	yes, absent harm (41-21-102)	if family member is a potential identifiable victim
Missouri Mo. Ann. Stat. §630-140 (West Supp. 1998)	X			yes	extent necessary to make a claim		if necessary to carry out duties; patient absent without consent	yes (630.110)	

Montana Mont. Code Ann. §53-21-166(mh); 50-16-529 (general)	X	qualified professional	extent necessary to make a claim		extent required by law (50-16-530)	absent harm (50-16-541; 542)	unless patient has instructed otherwise (50-16-29[4])
Nebraska Neb. Rev. Stat. §83-109 (1996)	X			reasonably identifiable victim (71-1,336)			
Nevada Nev. Rev. Stat. Ann. §433A. 360 (Michie 1996)	X	yes	extent necessary to make a claim		fraud inquiries (629.061)	yes (629.061)	
New Hampshire N.H. Rev. Stat. Ann. §135-C:19a (1996)	X	limited info. attempts to get consent					diagnosis, medications, and related info when family is caregiver
New Jersey N.J. Stat. Ann. §30:4–24-3 (West 1997)	X	X					patient's current medical condition

(continued)

State mental health confidentiality law provisions *(continued)*

State	Mental health law? Yes	No	Consent form detailed?	Provider access?	Payer access?	Danger to third party or self?	Law enforcement access?	Client access?	Family access?
New Mexico N.Mex. Stat. Ann. §43-1-19 (Michie 1993)	X		X		yes, with some limits	clear, imminent risk to self or others		unless not in patient's best interest	
New York N.Y. Laws §34A33.13 (McKinney 1996)	X			provider in approved local or unified service plan	yes	serious or imminent danger to third party	serious or imminent danger to third party; identifying data in criminal investigation	unless harm (33.16)	some access (33.16)
North Carolina N.C. Gen. Stat. §122c-52– 122C-56 (1996)	X			yes		imminent danger to client or third party or likelihood of crime		unless harm (122C-52)	with consent, diagnosis, prognosis, and medications, (122C-56); status changes without consent
North Dakota N.Dak. Cent. Code §25-03.1-43 (Michie Supp. 1997)	X			with consent	to extent necessary to perform functions		crime on premises		

Ohio Ohio Rev. Code Ann. §5122.31 (Anderson Supp. 1997)	X		yes, some limits on types of info	necessary medical information to insurers			unless clear treatment reasons	yes, absent patient objection
Oklahoma Okla. Stat. Ann. §43A-1-109 (West Supp. 1998) plan	X		qualified service agreement				with consent of treater or by court order	diagnosis, prognosis, medication; treatment
Oregon Or. Rev. Stat. §192.515–192.517 (1996)	X							
Pennsylvania 50 Pa. Cons. Stat. Ann. 7111; 4602 (Purdon Supp. 1998)	X		yes (4602)					
Rhode Island R.I. Gen. Laws §40.1-5-25–40.1-5-30 (1997)	X	yes (5-37)	yes	to extent necessary for aid, insurance, or medical assistance	if third party is endangered (5-37)	if patient has disappeared		diagnosis, medication, side effects; with patient consent

(continued)

State mental health confidentiality law provisions *(continued)*

State	Mental health law? Yes	No	Consent form detailed?	Provider access?	Payer access?	Danger to third party or self?	Law enforcement access?	Client access?	Family access?
South Carolina S.C. Code Ann. §44-22-100 (Law Co-op Supp. 1997)	X						when furthering welfare of patient or family	unless detrimental to patient (44-22-110)	current medical condition
South Dakota S.Dak. Codified Laws Ann. §27A-12-26 (1992; 1998 Supp.)	X			yes	yes		state attorney or attorney general for crime on premises	unless detrimental to client or confidential material, from another (27A-12-26.1)	admission or discharge status (27A-12-34)
Tennessee Tenn. Code Ann. §33-3-104(10) (LEXIS Supp. 1998)	X				third party payer (63-2-101)		crime on premises	applies to licensed professionals (A63-2-101)	current medical condition
Texas Tex. Health and Safety Code Ann. §611.002–611.008 (1992; West Supp. 1998)	X				those involved in paying or collecting fees	imminent harm to patient or others	imminent harm to patient or others	unless harm to patient (611.0045; 611.008)	

State								
Utah Utah Code Ann. §62A-12-247 (1997)	X							
Vermont Vt. Stat. Ann. title 18, §7103 (1987)	X							information concerning medical condition
Virginia Va. Code Ann. §37.1-225– 37.1-233 (Michie 1996)	X	for payer redisclosure (37.1-229)		patient who asks professional to submit a bill deemed to consent to certain disclosures (37.1-226)				access consistent with condition and sound treatment (37.1-84.1)
Washington Wash. Rev. Code Ann. §71.05.390 (mh); 70.02 (general) (West Supp. 1998)	X	yes (70.02.030)	in some circumstances (71.05.390; 70.02.050)	to extent necessary to make claim for aid, insurance or Medicaid (71.05.390)	threat to third party health or safety or if third party subject to harassment	status as patient; more info. upon sharing of need; third party in danger; patient absent without consent	yes (70.02.080)	oral communication permitted unless patient instructs otherwise (70.02.050)

(continued)

State	Mental health law? Yes	Mental health law? No	Consent form detailed?	Provider access?	Payer access?	Danger to third party or self?	Law enforcement access?	Client access?	Family access?
West Virginia W.Va Code §27-3-1; 27-5-9 (Michie 1992)	X			other health professional involved in treatment	Information required to certify that covered services were provided (27-5-9)	imminent injury to self or another			
Wisconsin Wis. Stat. Ann. §51-30 (West 1997)	X		yes	limitation on what types of providers can receive information	release to individuals for billing purposes		patient absent without consent; crime on premises; limited to identifying info.	access subject to restriction during treatment	prognosis diagnosis, and medications
Wyoming Wyo. Stat. §25-10-122 (mh); 35-2-605–35-2-616 (1997)	X		yes (35-2-607)	between mental health center, state hospital, and designated hospital (25-10-120)		to avoid imminent danger to self or others (35-2-609)	to extent required by law (35-2-609)	some limits (35-2-611; 35-2-612)	access unless patient instructs not to (35-2-609)

Index

Page numbers followed by "t" indicate tables; numbers followed by "n" indicate footnotes.

Abortion, parental notification of, 58
Accountability, 214
ACLU, *see* American Civil Liberties Union
Acting in reliance, 181
ADA, *see* Americans with Disabilities Act of 1990
Administrative simplification, 136–138
Adolescents
  with HIV/AIDS, 161–162
  and identity formation, 56
  see also Children
Alcohol/drug patients, 173–192
  child abuse/neglect and, 187–188
  disclosures about
    guidelines for, 178–191
    questions concerning, 179
    without consent, 107, 189
  legislation concerning, 96, 106–108
  medical emergencies with, disclosures during, 189
  medical records of
    court orders for, 185–187
    implicit versus explicit disclosure of, 177–178
    justice system and, 184–185
    refusal to disclose, 176–177
  patient-identifying information and, 189
  privacy of, notification of, 175
  qualified service organization agreement and, 191
  research programs and, 190–191
  stigma of, 174–175
  treatment programs for
    audits/evaluations of, 190–191
    confidentiality within, 188–189
    criminal behavior during, 189–190

definition of, 106n, 177
  written consent and, 180–185
    proper format for, 180
    requirements of, 180–183
American Civil Liberties Union (ACLU), poll on privacy, 8
American Medical Association, Code of Medical Ethics of, 91
American Psychiatric Association
  Committee for Privacy and Law of (or other preposition), 39
  on depression, 79
  and legislation, 13
American Psychological Association
  ethical principles of, 92
  Office on AIDS, 161
  on suicide, 168
Americans with Disabilities Act (ADA) of 1990 (PL 101-336), 2, 93, 108–109
  employment in, 201
  legal aid and, 43
  penalties in, 26
  and privacy of children, 51
Assisted suicide, 160, 168
Audits, 22–24, 117, 133
Autonomy, 66, 82, 94

Background checks on gun purchases, 15
Balanced Budget Act of 1997, 134n–135n
Bellotti v. Baird, 58
Blue Cross of California, 201
Bork, Robert, 193–194
Brady Handgun Violence Prevention Act, 15
Brandeis, Louis, 48
Breach of confidentiality, 110

Breach of fiduciary duty, 110

Canada, 130
Case examples, 77–78
Center for Public Integrity, The,
    194–195
Charter Orlando Hospital South, 26
Child abuse/neglect
  and alcohol/drug patients,
    187–188
  disclosure and, 104, 205
Children, 47–70
  and autonomy, 66
  custody of, 60
  and development of self, 55–56
  dignity of, 54–55
  privacy of,
    developmental perspective on,
      51–52
    family involvement and, 67
    importance of, 199
    institutions and, 54
    interested parties in, 47–48
    legal protection of, 60–62
    legal significance of, 56–59
    limitation of access to records
      and, 65
    in Nebraska, 62n
    need for standardization of, 64
    parties interested in, 49–51
    public policy concerning,
      62–65
    in school, 50–51, 58–59
    scope of interests in, 53–55
    self-fulfilling prophecies and,
      52
    treatment-related concerns of,
      75–76
  treatment for
    financial responsibility for, 62
    refusal of, 61n
    in schools, 63
  written consent of, 181–182
Cigna, 79
Clinical issues, 71–89, 134
Clinical training, privacy issues in,
    41–42
Clinton administration, 15, 65, 112,
    147
Code of Medical Ethics of Ameri-
    can Medical Association, 91

Coding of medical records, 141–142
Coercion, family therapy and, 41
Committee for Privacy and Law of
    American Psychiatric
    Association, 39
Communication, families and,
    35–37
Competence, 21
  and informed consent, 213
  and written consent, 182
Computer-based patient record
    (CPR), 138
Computers, 130–131, 143–144, 148,
    151–152
  see also Electronic medical
    records
Condit, Gary, 128, 129n
Confidentiality
  definition of, 96–97
    for consumer, 7
  and distinction from privacy,
    53–55
  exceptions to, 97–106
  purposes of, 53
  tiers of, 151, 151n, 211–212
  see also Privacy
Confidentiality of Individually-
    Identifiable Health
    Information, 81, 83
Confidentiality of Individually-
    Identifiable Health
    Information . . ., 13
"Confidentiality of Records,"
    173–174
Consent
  to disclosure, 97–99
  see also Informed consent;
    Written consent
Consent forms, use of, 183–184
Constitution, privacy protection in,
    56–57
Consumer
  access to own records of, 21–22,
    39, 105–106
  definition of privacy and confi-
    dentiality for, 7
  perspective on privacy of, 5–32
  respect for, 26–27
  rights of, 16–17
Consumer rights protection, 13
Consumerism
  definition of, 12–13

versus paternalism, 12–14
Content areas, distinguishing, 37–38
Contumelia, 197
Convention on the Rights of the
     Child, 57–58, 67
Costs of health care, 72
     containment of, 83, 133, 206
     and federal legislation, 148–149
Court orders, 185–187
     denial of, 186–187
CPR, *see* Computer-based patient
     record
Criminal investigations
     court orders and, 185–187
     disclosure and, 183–184, 205
Culture, privacy and, 42–43

*Darlene Vasconcellos v. Cybex
     International,* 86
Data protection, 128, 196–197
Deceased patients, privacy of,
     182–183
Defamation, 110
Degradation rituals, 54
Deinstitutionalization, families
     and, 35, 40–41
Delta Airlines, 201
Department of Health and Human
     Services (DHHS), 92,
     112–113, 132, 137–138
Depression
     characteristics of, 200
     screening for, 79
     treatment program for, 73–74
Deus Machine, The (Ovellette), 18
Developmental psychology of
     privacy, 55–56
DHHS, *see* Department of Health
     and Human Services
Digital signatures, 24, 146
Disclosure
     about alcohol/drug patients, 107
     of child abuse/neglect, 104,
          187–188, 205
     consent to, 97–99
     court orders for family law and,
          185–187
     for criminal investigations,
          183–184
     federal confidentiality rules,
          requirements for, 176–178

harmful results of, 199–202
     of HIV/AIDS, *see* HIV/AIDS
     implicit versus explicit, 177–178
     to justice system, 184–185
     to legal counsel, 104
     limitations of, 211–212
     during medical emergencies,
          116–117, 189
     in private sectors, 74
     to qualified service organization,
          191
     for quality control, 100–101
     range of, 34
     reasons for, 97–106
     and redisclosure, 183
     risk management and, 38
     and sexually transmitted
          diseases, 204–205
     suicide and, 200
     for third party protection,
          102–103
     unauthorized use of, 131
     in workplace, 79, 201
Discrimination, 93–94
Disease management, access to
          individual cases by, 203
Doctor–patient privilege, 198
Doctor–patient relationship, trust
     in, 9, 94, 199, 212
Drivers Privacy Protection,
     150–151
Drug testing
     and federal confidentiality rules,
          176
     in schools, 59
Drugs, *see* Alcohol/drug patients

Education of families, 36–37
Edwards, Don, 188
Electronic Communications
     Privacy Act of 1986
     (PL 99-508), 184
Electronic medical records, 5, 79–80
     access to, ease of, 22
     option out of, 21
     problems with, 11–12
     removal of data from, 20, 24–25
     risks with, 143–144
     security of, 215
     and zones of privacy, 211
Ellsberg, Daniel, 15

Emergencies, *see* Disclosures
Emotional distress, 110
Employers, access to records by, 132–133
Encryption of medical records, 142–143, 149
Entwined identity, 34–35
Equifax Harris Consumer Privacy Survey (1993), 8
Ethical and Legal and Social Implications Program of Human Genome Project, 202
Ethical Rules, 166
Ethics, 91–125
   of American Psychological Association, 92
   and medical research, 8
Ethnicity, 42–43
   and mental illness, 35
European Union, privacy directive of, 209

Fair Credit Reporting Act (PL 104-208), 194–195
Fair Health Information Practices Act of 1997, 129, 140, 148, 150*n*
Fair Housing Amendments Act of 1988 (PL 100-430), 93
Fair information practices, 128–129, 128*n*–129*n*
Fairfax County law enforcement, 173–174
Families, 33–46
   access to records by, 99–100, 111, 117
   as caregivers, information needed by, 37–38
   communication with, 35–37
   and contact with patient, 40
   and content areas of privacy, 37–38
   culture of, 42–43
   and deinstitutionalization, 35, 40–41
   education of, 36–37
   and entwined identity, 34–35
   and privacy of children, 67
   see also Parents
Family law, court orders for disclosure and, 185, 187

Family relationships, aspects of, 33–35
Family therapy, 41–42
Faxing medical records, security of, 23
Federal Alcohol and Substance Abuse Law, 106–108
Federal confidentiality rules
   definitions in, 176–178
   notification of, 175
   requirements for disclosure, 176–178
Federal legislation, 112–113, 134–135, 147–152
   preemption of, 118–120
   proposals for, 114–118
Federal mental health confidentiality law, 106–110
Federal Rules of Evidence, 109
Federal substance abuse law, 209–210
Fiduciary duty, breach of, 110
Final Report of the Legislative Survey of State Confidentiality Laws with Specific Emphasis on HIV and Immunizations, The, 23–24
Financial services industry, access to information in, 194–195
Fingerprint identification technology, 24
FOIA, *see* Freedom of Information Act of 1964
Foster, Vince, 199–200
Fourth Amendment, 58–59, 66
Fraud, prevention of, 133, 206
Freedom of Information Act (FOIA) of 1964 (PL 89-554), 108

Gender discrimination, 59*n*
General Accounting Office, 133*n*
Genetic antidiscrimination bill, 201
Genetic information, misuse of, 201–202
Genetic testing, 200–201
Government
   access to records by, 132–133
   and medical privacy, 15
Greek law, privacy in, 197
Griswold v. Connecticut, 56
Guardian *ad litem,* 60

Gun purchases, background checks on, 15

Haines, Don, 19
Harvard Law Review, 127, 197
Harvard Pilgrim Health Care, 150*n*
Health care costs, *see* Costs of healthcare
Health care system, changes in, 2
Health care trustee, 115
Health Information Modernization and Security Act, 195
Health Insurance Portability and Accountability Act (HIPAA) of 1996 (PL 104-191), 18–19, 92, 112–113, 134, 136–138, 137*n*, 196
Hippocratic Oath, 71, 91–125
HIV/AIDS, 157–171
    adolescents with, 161–162
    disclosure of, 204
        decision-making process in, 164
        guidelines for, 166
        premature, 163
        societal versus individual rights and, 165–166
    duty to treat, 158
    history of, 157–158
    in institutions, 165
    in prison population, 164–165
    and risk to others, case examples of, 159–160
    stigma of, 158
    suicide and, 160, 167–169
    testing, 159
    unsafe sex and, 162–167
Hobson, David, 195
Hodgson v. Minnesota, 58
Hudson v. Palmer, 59
Human Genome Project, 75, 202
Humanistic approach, 12, 26–27

Identity
    entwined, 34–35
    formation of, 55–56
In re Commissioner of Social Services v. David R.S., 178
In re Romance M, 187
In re Stephen F., 187

Individually identifiable health information, 138–144
    definition of, 113
Informed consent, 20–21, 81–84, 97–99, 212–213
    competence and, 213
    factors in, 20–21
    and family therapy, 41
    requirements for, 115–118, 213
    research and, 83–84
    third-party payer and, 82
    see also Written consent
Injuria, 197
Institute of Medicine, 75, 95
Institutional Review Boards (IRB), 25–26, 203
Institutions
    HIV/AIDS in, 165–166
    intrusiveness of treatment in, 54
    see also Deinstitutionalization
Insurance, inability to obtain, 201–202
Insurance Bureau of Canada, 130
International Covenant on Civil and Political Rights, 57
Inviolate personality, 198
IRB, *see* Institutional Review Boards

Jaffee v. Redmond, 73, 85, 105, 109, 198
JCAHO, *see* Joint Commission on Accreditation of Healthcare Organizations
Jeanette "A." v. Condon, 176
Joint Commission on Accreditation of Healthcare Organizations (JCAHO), 27
Joyner v. Dumpson, 60
Justice system, 85–86
    disclosure to, 104–105, 184–185
Juvenile Justice Standards, 61–62

Kennedy-Kassebaum, *see* Health Insurance Portability and Accountability Act of 1996

Law enforcement agencies
    access to records by, 84–85, 103–104, 116, 133, 206–208

Law enforcement agencies—
  continued
  and alcohol/drug records,
    173–174
Laws, *see* Legislation
Lawsuits, reasons for, 110
Lee v. Corregedore, 103
Legal counsel, disclosure to, 104
Legal guardians, 60
Legislation, 2, 13, 15, 91–125, 216
  in European Union, 209
  federal, *see* Federal legislation
  federal versus state versus indi-
    vidual, 147–152
  concerning HIV/AIDS, 162–163
  lack of, 134*n*–135*n*, 134–136
  options for, 208–214
  penalties of, 26, 214
  problems with, 110–112
  state, *see* State legislation
"Live and Let Live" (ACLU), 8
Longitudinal medical records, 95
Los Angeles County-USC Psychi-
    atric Outpatient Clinic,
    73–74
Los Angeles Outpatient Clinic,
    78–79
Lovelace Health Systems, 79

Managed care, 2, 72, 98
  access to records in, 5–7, 79
  and cost containment, 83
  and refusal of treatment, 74
  resistance to change of, 10
Master patient access mediator, 146
Mature minor rule, 60–61
Medical advances, 75, 200–202
Medical emergencies, disclosures
    during, 116–117, 189
Medical Privacy in the Age of New
    Technologies Act of 1997,
    139–140, 140*n*–141*n*, 151*n*
Medical products, sales of, 133*n*
Medical records, 78–81
  access to, 7–12
    benefits of, 6
    by consumers, 21–22, 39,
      105–106
    by employers, 132–133
    by families, 99–100, 111, 117,
      206–208
  by government, 132–133
  by justice system, 85–86,
    184–185
  by law enforcement agencies,
    84–85, 103–104, 116, 133,
    206–208
  by managed care, 79
  by providers, 98, 111, 115–116
  for research, 101, 117
  risks of, 6
  by third party, 22, 78–79, 99,
    111, 115–116, 132–133, 206
coding of, 141–142
data collection guidelines for, 23
disclosure of, *see* Disclosure
distribution of, 22–24
encryption of, 142–143, 149
information contained in, 80
linkage of, 146
longitudinal, 95
nonidentifiable, 139–141
ownership of, 10–11, 17–18,
    38–42
on paper, 130
person-driven protections of,
    19–27
protected, 114–115
purpose of, 78
removal of data from, 24–25
security of, 10, 22–24
sensitivity of, special treatment
    of, 210–211
storage of, 22–24
theft of, 130
unique identifier on, 24, 95,
    106–107, 144–145, 195–196
users of, 132–134
uses of, 95, 132–134
see also Electronic medical
    records
Medical Records Confidentiality
    Act, 142
Medicare, 109
Mental health treatment notes, 151
Mental illness
  ethnlcity and, 35
  privacy issues in, 9–10
  public opinion of, 43–44
  stigma of, 1, 9, 93–94
Model Mental Health Confidential-
    ity Statute, proposal of,
    121–123

Model State Public Health Privacy
Project, 204, 214
Morgan v. Fairfield Family Counseling Center, 102

National Alliance for the Mentally
Ill, Office of Homeless and
Missing Persons of, 39
National Association of Social
Workers on end-of-life issues, 168
National Coalition of Mental Health
Professionals and Consumers, Inc., 77
National Committee on Vital and
Health Statistics (NCVHS), 9,
83, 112–114, 132, 144, 144*n*
on review boards, 16
Subcommittee on Privacy and
Confidentiality, 113, 137,
138*n*
National Health Care Data Network,
75
National Research Council, 143
National standards, 111
NCVHS, *see* National Committee
on Vital and Health Statistics
Nebraska, privacy of children in,
62*n*
Negligence, 110
New Jersey v. T.L.O., 58–59
New York City Methadone Maintenance Treatment Program,
174
New York Statewide Planning and
Research Cooperative System (SPARCS), 139*n*
Newman, Robert, 174
Next of kin, disclosures to, 117
Nonidentifiability, tests for, 140
see also Medical records
Non-personally identifiable information, 138–144
access to, 203
Nothing Sacred: The Politics of Privacy, 194
Nuremberg Code, 14

Office of Homeless and Missing
Persons, 39

Office on AIDS, American Psychological Association, 161
Olmstead v. United States, 48
Option out, of electronic record
system, 21
Outcome studies, 14
Outcome-based decision making, 7
Oversight, 117
and disclosure, 100–101
Ownership of medical records,
10–11, 17–18, 38–42

Panel on Confidentiality and Data
Access of the Committee on
National Statistics, 140*n*
Paper records, abuse of, 130
Parental notification, abortion and,
58
Parents
and custody of children, 60
and privacy of children, 49–50,
67
see also Families
Paternalism, consumerism versus,
12–14
Patient tracking, 7
Patient-identifying information of
alcohol/drug patients, 189
Patients
self-revelations by, 71–72
see also Consumer
Penalties, 214
of breach of privacy, 26
Performance measurement, access
to individual cases by, 203
Personal health identifier, 24, 95,
106–107, 144–145, 195–196
Personally identifiable information,
138–144, 203
Person-driven protections of medical records, 19–27
PL 89-554, *see* Freedom of Information Act of 1964
PL 93-579, *see* Privacy Act of 1974
PL 99-508, *see* Electronic Communications Privacy Act of
1986
PL 100-430, *see* Fair Housing
Amendments Act of 1988
PL 100-618, *see* Video Privacy Protection Act of 1988

PL 101-336, *see* Americans with
Disabilities Act of 1990
PL 102-321, *see* Public Health Services Act
PL 104-191, *see* Health Insurance
Portability and Accountability Act of 1996
PL 104-208, *see* Fair Credit Reporting Act
*Planned Parenthood of Central
Missouri v. Danforth,* 58
Politics, medical privacy and, 15
Practice guidelines, 36–37
Presumed consent, 213
Prime, C.J., 79
Principles for the Protection of persons with Mental Illness and the Improvement of Mental Health Care, 58
Prisons
HIV/AIDS in, 164–165
privacy in, 59
Privacy
concept of, 48
definition for consumer of, 7
developmental psychology of, 55–56
and distinction from confidentiality, 53–55
importance of, 196–202
for children, 199
limits to
and cost containment, 206
and family access, 206–208
and fraud prevention, 206
importance of, 202–208
and law enforcement access, 206–208
protection of others and, 205–206
public health and, 204
and quality of care, 203–204
and politics, 15
public and child, 48
reasons for wanting, 198–199
right to, 94
development of idea of, 197–198
State laws and, 219–232
and treatment-related concerns
of adults, 73–75
of children, 75–76
values underlying, 93–96
integrity of, 95–96
violation of, results of, 199–202
zones of, 62, 95, 211–212
see also Confidentiality
Privacy Act of 1974 (PL 93-579), 108, 127, 135
Private sector, disclosure in, 74
Privileged information, 104–105
Program evaluation, disclosure and, 100–101
Protected health information, definition of, 140
Protected health information subfile, 151n
Provider networks, 98
Providers
access to records by, 111, 115–116
and child privacy, 47
disclosure to, 98
Psychodynamic psychotherapy, 36
Public, child privacy and, 48
Public health reporting, 101, 118, 134, 204
Public Health Services Act (PL 102-321), 106
Public opinion polls, 8–9, 92

Qualified service organization agreement, 191
Quality control, and disclosure, 100–101
Quality of care, limits to privacy and, 203–204

Reasonable basis to believe test, 140
"Records, Computers, and the Rights of Citizens," 19
Redisclosure, written prohibition on, 183
Redmond v. Jaffee, 86
Reimbursement, 99
Research
access to records for, 7–8, 13–14, 101, 117, 203–204
on alcohol/drug patients, 190–191
denied to public access, 14
ethical questions in, 8
informed consent and, 83–84

Review boards, 25–26
    access to records by, 203
    information needed by, 80–81
    NCVHS on, 16
Revocation of consent, 181
Right to privacy, development of
        idea of, 197–198
Risk management, disclosure and
        38
Roe v. Wade, 57
Roman law, privacy in, 197

Schall v. Martin, 59
Schools
    drug testing in, 59
    mental health services in, 63
    privacy of children in, 50–51,
        58–59
Scott, Patricia, 201
Security, 131*n*, 131–132
    of medical records, 10, 22–24, 215
        future of, 24
        and sensitivity of information,
            62–63, 210–211
            unique identifier and, 24, 95,
                106–107, 144–145, 195–196
Security audits, 22–24, 117, 133
Self
    integrity of, 199
    in relation to society, 55–56
Self-esteem, intrusive treatment,
        and 54
Self-fulfilling prophecies, privacy
        of children, and 52
Self-revelations during treatment,
        71–72
Sensitivity of information, security
        and, 62–63, 210–211
Service Employees International
        Union, 201
Service organization, definition of,
        191
Sex, unsafe, HIV/AIDS and,
        162–167
Sexually transmitted diseases,
        disclosure and, 204–205
Shalala, Donna E., 26, 81, 83–84,
        113, 202–203
Signature for written consent,
        181–182
Social Security Act, 134*n*–135*n*

Social security number (SSN), 145,
        145*n*
    access to, 194–195
    and security of records, 24
SPARCS, *see* New York Statewide
        Planning and Research
        Cooperative System
SSN, *see* Social security number
Standards, 136–138, 148–149
    for mental health and substance
        abuse, integration of,
        120–121
    national, 111
    for privacy of children, 64
State laws, privacy and, 219–232
State legislation, 135, 147–152,
        219–232
    concerning privacy, 96–106
    diversity of, 149
    preemption of, 118–120
    variation in, 209
State mental health confidentiality
        laws, 96–106
State v. Friedman, 176
State v. Rollinson, 186
Stigma
    of HIV/AIDS, 158
    of mental illness, 1, 93–94
Storytelling in therapeutic process,
        71–72
Styron, William, 200
Subcommittee on Privacy and Con-
        fidentiality of National Com-
        mittee on Vital and Health
        Statistics, 113, 137, 138*n*
Suicide, 103, 160
    disclosure and, guidelines for,
        168
    HIV/AIDS and, 167–169
    and risk of disclosure, 200
Supreme Court, 56–57, 109–110
Surrogate consent, 21

Talmud, privacy in, 197
*Tarasoff v. Regents of the Univer-
        sity of California,* 38, 102,
        163–164, 205
Teachers, mental health of children
        and, 63
Technology, 127–156
    definition of, 129–130

Technology—*continued*
  and medical records, 5, 95
    see also Electronic medical
      records
  and privacy, 198
Terminal illness, suicide and,
    167–169
Theft, of medical records, 130
Therapeutic process, storytelling
    in, 71–72
Therapist-client privilege, 198
Third-party payers
  and access to records, 22, 78–79,
    99, 111, 115–116, 132–133,
    206
    for alcohol/drug treatment, 181
  and child privacy, 47
  informed consent and, 82
  security and, 23–24
Third-party reviewers, information
    needed by, 80–81
Tiers of confidentiality, 151, 151*n*,
    211–212
Total Quality Management (TQM),
    13
TQM, *see* Total Quality Manage-
    ment
Transference, 36
Trauma, self-revelations and, 71–72
Treatment programs
  for alcohol/drug patients, crimi-
    nal behavior during,
    189–190
  confidentiality within, 188–189
  intrusiveness of, 53–54
  refusal of, 74
    by children, 61*n*
    fear of disclosure and, 9, 76–78
Treatment-related privacy concerns
  of adults, 73–75
  of children, 75–76
  Trust in doctor-patient
    relationship, 9, 94, 199, 212
Turner, Jacob, 201

Uniform Health-Care Information
    Act, 121*n*
Unique identifier on medical
    records, 24, 95, 106–107,
    144–145, 195–196
United States v. Graham, 187
United States v. Smith, 187
Unsafe sex, HIV/AIDS and, 162–167
  disclosure and, 167
Utilization review, access to indi-
    vidual cases by, 203

Velaquez, Nydia, 6
*Veronia School District 47J v.
    Acton,* 59
Video Privacy Protection Act of
    1988 (PL 100-618), 135*n*,
    193–194, 196
Violation, 198
Virtual systems, 23

Watergate, 15
Whalen v. Roe, 109
WHO, *see* World Health
    Organization
*Whyte v. Connecticut Mutual Life
    Insurance Co.,* 182
*Williams ex re. Williams v.
    Ellington,* 59
Workplace, disclosures in, 74, 79,
    201
World Health Organization (WHO),
    42–43
Written consent
  for alcohol/drug treatment,
    180–185
  competence and, 182
  of minors, 181–182
  revocation of, 181
  use of, 183–184
  see also Informed consent

Zones of privacy, 95, 211–212